HERE

BE

DRAGONS

HERE BE

ONE MAN'S QUEST TO
MAKE HEALTHCARE MORE
ACCESSIBLE AND AFFORDABLE

BE
DRAGONS

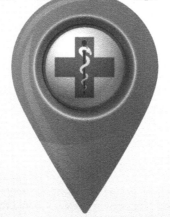

WEB GOLINKIN

Forbes | Books

Published by Forbes Books, Charleston, South Carolina.
An imprint of Advantage Media Group.

Forbes Books is a registered trademark, and the Forbes Books colophon is a trademark of Forbes Media, LLC.

Printed in the United States of America.

10 9 8 7 6 5 4 3 2 1

ISBN: 978-1-95588-454-9 (Hardcover)
ISBN: 978-1-95588-453-2 (eBook)

Library of Congress Control Number: 2023917329

Cover design by Lance Buckley.
Layout design by David Taylor.

Since 1917, Forbes has remained steadfast in its mission to serve as the defining voice of entrepreneurial capitalism. Forbes Books, launched in 2016 through a partnership with Advantage Media, furthers that aim by helping business and thought leaders bring their stories, passion, and knowledge to the forefront in custom books. Opinions expressed by Forbes Books authors are their own. To be considered for publication, please visit **books.Forbes.com**.

To the many talented and dedicated teammates who have joined me in this quest, and to Allison, Jeb, and Will, who have been my inspiration and support system.

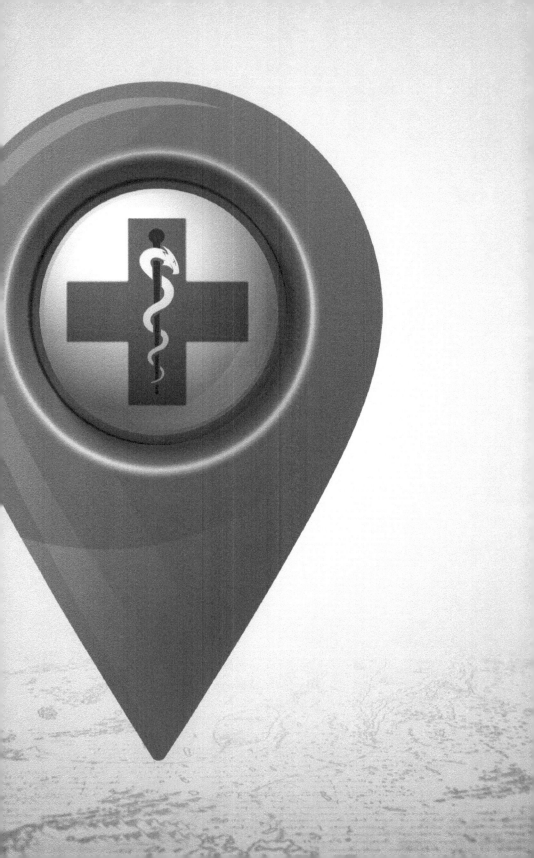

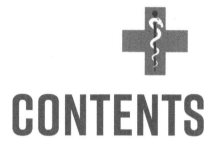

CONTENTS

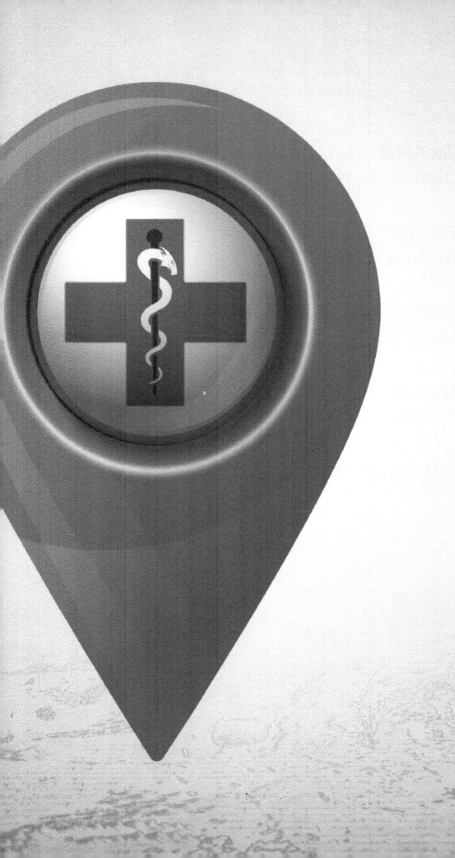

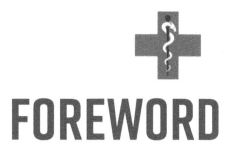

FOREWORD

This book is the personal story of an individual of astonishing passion and tenacity who has spent the last three decades trying to make health information and care more accessible to the average consumer. It is also a story of creativity and resilience in the face of an intractable medical establishment and many other seemingly insurmountable obstacles.

Web Golinkin weaves us through his upbringing, education, and early years, followed by the discovery of his passion for healthcare that has been the focus of his illustrious but unusual career. The bulk of this book is devoted to the world of on-demand medicine, which until the introduction of urgent care and retail clinics—that Web helped to pioneer—was the exclusive domain of hospital emergency departments. The more cost-effective models Web developed for delivering routine acute episodic and preventive care have been embraced by consumers with great enthusiasm due to their superior accessibility and affordability—but retailers, third-party payors, government regulators, and many physician groups did not initially see the light.

The idea that Web and a small number of other retail medicine pioneers had twenty years ago seemed so elegantly simple: to open limited-service healthcare clinics inside conveniently located retail outlets and staff them with nurse practitioners and physician assistants rather than physicians. Make basic healthcare more accessible and affordable, and in the process create a "portal" into the nation's immense and absurdly complex healthcare system. However, as one veteran of retail medicine once told me, "In healthcare, simple is hard."

Once the external obstacles to success had been neutralized (though certainly not eliminated), Web and others had to figure out how to turn retail and urgent care clinics into sustainable businesses. While these clinics tended to thrive during the cough-cold-flu season, patient volumes tapered significantly during the spring and summer months. Many clinic operators ultimately failed because of this, but Web and his team were able to survive and eventually prosper by offering more immunizations, physicals, and other preventive services with year-round demand and significant patient and public health benefits, including an innovative weight management program.

But the one thing that has enabled Web to succeed in effecting transformative change in healthcare—while many other high-profile entrepreneurs and organizations have failed—is his relentless focus on the healthcare patient as a customer. Without a medical background himself, Web has viewed healthcare from the perspective of the customer, concentrating on the ultimate goal of earning consistently high Net Promoter Scores (over 85) and the key role of supporting his companies' patient-facing team members in their efforts to achieve them.

In addition to overcoming resistance from the medical establishment and other constituencies that were essential to his survival and success, as well as meeting the challenges of creating a new business model, Web has had to grapple with many unpredictable events that would have defeated all but the most committed and creative individuals, including financing challenges during the Great Recession, the COVID-19 pandemic, a major financing that failed on the day it was supposed to close, the acquisition of a major investor by an unsupportive new owner, a high-profile investor who pulled out after deciding that revolutionizing healthcare was too difficult to pursue, and even the seemingly unwarranted interference by the Federal Trade Commission (FTC) in an acquisition that could have reduced healthcare costs.

Many skillful entrepreneurs, sophisticated private equity firms, large hospital systems, and multi-billion-dollar companies like Amazon and Walmart are still trying to figure out how to make our nation's $4 trillion healthcare system more accessible and affordable, thus far with limited success. What Web and the small number of other individuals who essentially invented what we now refer to as retail medicine have done against all odds represents one of the few bright spots in this effort.

Not only have Web and others made basic healthcare more accessible and affordable to millions of consumers directly through their clinics, but they have also indirectly forced many of the traditional healthcare players to be more efficient and consumer-centric. And in the course of Web's challenging journey, he has also built strong teams and cultures, so you will find many hard-earned leadership lessons in this book that apply to any company in any industry.

Web is one of the individuals who gets credit for this amazing transformation: more transparent pricing, more accessible care, higher patient satisfaction, lower costs, and simplified workflows. What he has achieved is a classic example of what the late Clayton Christiansen famously referred to as "disruptive innovation."

Tom Charland
Founder and retired CEO
Merchant Medicine, LLC

Tom Charland is the founder and former CEO of Merchant Medicine, LLC, a leading healthcare research and management consulting firm that was acquired in 2020 by Urgent Care Partners to form UCP Merchant Medicine. Tom introduced the concept of ConvUrgentCare® (pronounced convergent care), the mingling of operating tactics from convenient care (retail clinics), urgent care, work site clinics, primary care, and telemedicine. He started the annual Merchant Medicine Strategy Symposium, a conference that covers the on-demand medicine industry. He has been quoted on this subject in the The Wall Street Journal, Forbes, *the* New York Times, Chicago Tribune, *the* Boston Globe, Fox News, Bloomberg, *and other media outlets.*

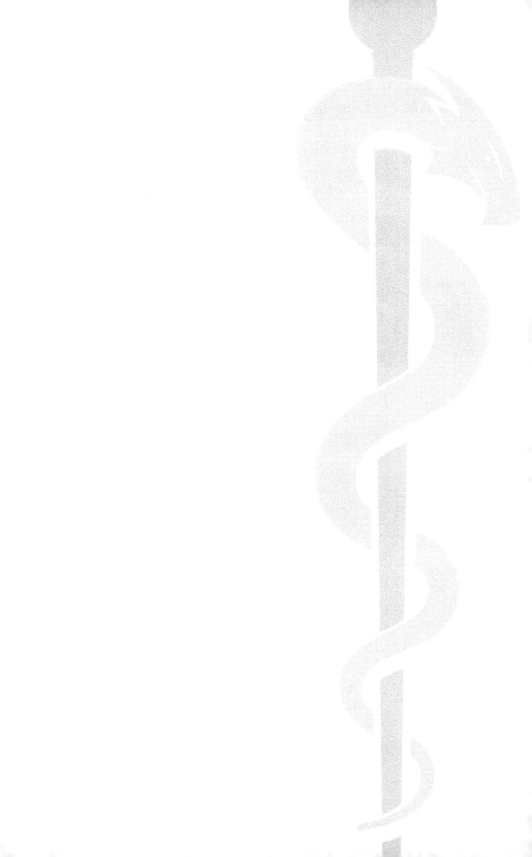

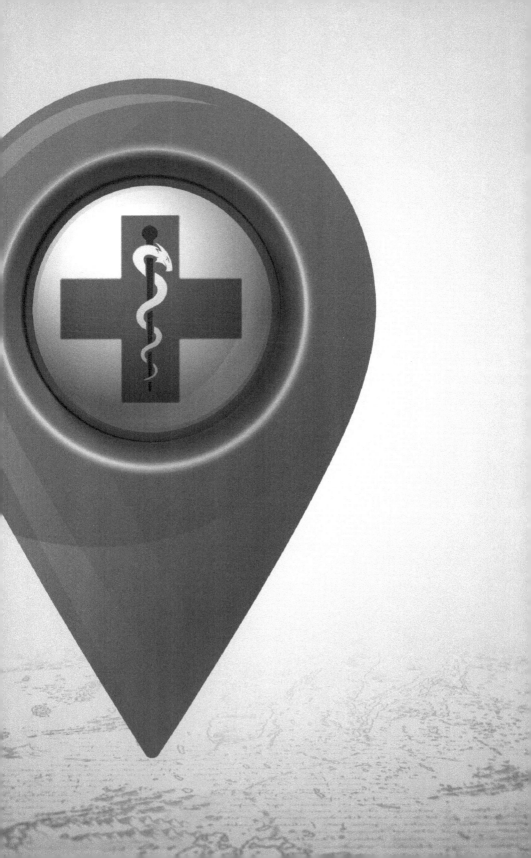

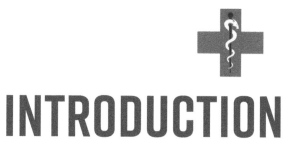

INTRODUCTION

Healthcare is America's largest industry. It currently represents over $4 trillion in annual spending and accounts for about one-fifth of the entire U.S. economy, and annual healthcare spending is expected to grow to more than $7 trillion by 2031.[1] It is also America's largest employer with more than twenty-one million people working in the healthcare industry.[2] In many cities across America, the local hospital or healthcare system is among the largest employers.

The United States also spends more on healthcare than any other major industrialized country but gets less. According to a recent report by the Commonwealth Fund, comparing the United States to ten other large countries, America spends more on healthcare than any

---

1   Sean P. Keehan, et al., "National Health Expenditure Projections 2022-31," *Health Affairs: Medicare, Cancer & More* 42, no. 7 (July 2023), https://www.healthaffairs.org/doi/10.1377/hlthaff.2023.00403.

2   Earlene K.P. Powell, "Healthcare Still Largest U.S. Employer," U.S. Census Bureau, October 14, 2020, https://www.census.gov/library/stories/2020/10/health-care-still-largest-united-states-employer.html.

other by a wide margin, both as a percentage of the overall economy and on a per capita basis. And yet when ranking these large countries according to five categories—one of which is "access to care"—the United States ranks dead last. (No pun intended, although as it turns out the United States is also last in life expectancy.)[3]

Why is that? The U.S. healthcare system is large, complex, and highly regulated, with many vested interests that are resistant to change, even though our system is failing us in many ways. It is generally effective at managing a relatively small number of highly complex cases but ineffective in managing a much larger number of routine cases that negatively impact quality of life and productivity and can become life-threatening and expensive if not treated promptly. The system also struggles to provide the kind of preventive care that promotes and maintains public health—as we've seen recently with COVID-19.

More than thirty years ago, I set out to change that, initially by giving consumers easier access to the information they need to take charge of their own health (American Medical Communications and America's Health Network) and then to give them easier access to healthcare itself through the creation and operation of retail-based and urgent care clinics (RediClinic and FastMed). A substantial part of my career has been spent trying to figure out how to make the healthcare system more accessible and affordable. At times, what I've done has been driven by necessity but also because I had a vision of what I wanted to accomplish. Amid the successes, there have been many "near-death" experiences.

---

3   The Commonwealth Fund, "Mirror, Mirror 2021: Healthcare in the United States Compares to Other High Income Countries," August 4, 2021, https://www.commonwealthfund.org/publications/fund-reports/2021/aug/mirror-mirror-2021-reflecting-poorly.

Over time, I have founded and/or led multiple healthcare companies, taking each from one stage to the next in a tremendous set of adventures. Much of what I learned along the way you don't learn in business schools because frequently I was inventing these businesses while running them—building the plane while flying it, as they say. It has required a lot of hard work and no small number of sleepless nights, but I have survived and ultimately made a small dent in our nation's massive healthcare system mainly because I've been passionate about making it more accessible and affordable and blessed to have worked with many talented people who have been equally committed to this mission.

It took me a while to find this passion. I grew up in New York City and Long Island, the only child of older, working parents. My father, Joseph Golinkin, was fifty-five when I was born and had already fought in two world wars. My mother, Ruth Fowler, was forty. My father grew up in Chicago, one of seven children, and attended the Art Institute of Chicago for one year before being admitted to the U.S. Naval Academy. He graduated just in time to serve in World War I. After the war, he returned to his passion for art, creating oils, watercolors, drawings, and lithographs that recorded two of his favorite subjects: New York City and sports. He was awarded a gold medal for sporting art at the 1932 Olympics in Los Angeles, the last year awards were given in this category.

My father's art was exhibited internationally and is contained in many museum and private collections. In 1929, his New York scenes were featured in the book, *New York Is Like This*, and in 1941, his sports scenes were collected in the book *The American Sporting Scene* with text by *New York Times* sportswriter and commentator John Kieran. In my father's 1977 obituary in *Newsday*, Kieran said that Joseph Golinkin's paintings "cast such a spell over me that in my enthusiasm, I was driven to write a book around them."[4]

In 1941, my father was called back into active service in the U.S. Navy where he served with distinction, earning a Bronze Star, the Naval Reserve Medal with two stars, and the U.S. Victory Medal, eventually retiring in 1958 with the rank of rear admiral. As was typical of his generation, my father did not talk much about his life growing up or his experience during two world wars, but as I told *Newsday* in 1977: "He was incredibly disciplined and at the same time very sensitive. His most distinctive characteristic was the way he integrated his startlingly different careers."[5]

My mother grew up in California and, like me, was an only child. She went first to the University of California, Los Angeles (UCLA), and then to the University of Chicago, eventually volunteering to serve in World War II. She was in the first class of commissioned officers in the Women's Army Corps (WAC) and, after the war, retired as a major in the U.S. Army. She had many stories about how enlisted men would refuse to salute her because she was a woman. She was also a poster girl during the war, featured on a famous war bond poster showing a woman in military uniform holding an index finger to her lips above the caption "Silence Means Security." (If you Google "Silence Means Security," you'll see her poster!) My parents met after the war, married in 1949, and settled in Oyster Bay on the north shore of Long Island.

More than anything, my parents wanted me to have a great education, and I attended two prestigious private schools in K–12, where I was typically one of the least affluent kids in my class. Not that

---

4   "Joseph Golinkin, 80, Officer, Artist," *Newsday* (Nassau Edition, Hempstead, NY) September 9, 1977, p. 43.

5   "Joseph Golinkin, 80, Officer, Artist."

my parents were poor, but my father was still in the Navy and then was commandant of the Philadelphia Navy Yard, and my mother was an assistant publisher at *LIFE* magazine, where she was paid much less than her male colleagues. It was clear that my family didn't have the resources that many of my classmates enjoyed, but I always felt blessed and took to heart the admonition from Luke 12:48: "To whom much is given, much will be required."

For grade school, I went to St. Bernard's in New York City, which was a stuffy private school on the Upper East Side of Manhattan with a distinctively British flavor. I didn't like it much, but it gave me a great early education. My father would drive my mother and me from Long Island into the city every Monday morning, dropping me off at school and then my mother at the TIME-LIFE building on his way to Philadelphia. He would then reverse the trip on Friday afternoon.

My mother and I lived in a small, rent-controlled apartment in the city during the week. I was the only kid in my class whose mother had a job. The other mothers felt sorry for me, like I was missing something, but I never felt that way. My mother was doing interesting things, covering some of the most momentous events of the 1960s, from the Kennedy assassination to the Apollo astronauts. I loved visiting her at LIFE, which was in its heyday. Her colleagues were bright, energetic, committed to their work, and having an impact on the world.

Both my parents were that way. My father was passionate about his art, and he was equally passionate about his country and the Navy, but he never mixed the two. When he was in the Navy, he never painted. I asked him about that once, and his response was that his job in the Navy was to defend our country and that painting couldn't help with that. The Navy wanted him to paint battle scenes, but he refused, so they sent him off to captain destroyers and destroyer escorts in the

Mediterranean and Pacific. My mother was equally committed to her craft, the way most journalists are. I learned about the importance of passion, commitment, and making a contribution from my parents, each of whom served multiple terms as mayor of our local village later in their lives.

For high school, I went to St. George's, a private school in Newport, Rhode Island, which was where I started to find my footing. It was my father's painting that led me to St. George's. One of my father's favorite artistic subjects was sailing (the only place that his naval and artistic interests intersected), and he was in Newport painting the America's Cup races when he met a man named Norris "Norry" Hoyt, an avid sailor who reported on all the major sailing races over the radio. Norry had been the captain of the 1936 Yale swimming team and served on a PT boat during World War II. After the war, in 1946, Norry came to St. George's to teach English, where he stayed for twenty-nine years. My father introduced me to Norry, and he encouraged me to attend St. George's. Norry and my father ultimately collaborated on a book, *The Twelve Meter Challenges for the America's Cup*, published in 1977, just before my father passed away.

I performed well enough at St. George's to gain admission to Harvard. I had planned to do Navy Reserve Officers' Training Corps (NROTC) there, which would have provided a free education while allowing me to follow in my father's footsteps by serving in the military. Unfortunately, it was the same year, 1969, that Harvard canceled its ROTC programs amid protests over the Vietnam War. Once again, my parents scraped together everything they could to get me through college.

Harvard was challenging, and I was enjoying it, but it was a confusing time to be on college campuses, and without NROTC I wasn't sure what I wanted to do or even what I wanted to study. I had always had a fantasy about sailing around the world. And so—after riding a motorcycle more than 7,000 miles across the country the summer after my sophomore year—I just decided to do it. I told my parents that I wanted to take some time off from Harvard because I wasn't getting much out of it and felt like I was wasting their money, and they were quite understanding about it. Raising an only child as older parents, they were always conscious of making sure I was independent, not spoiled as some only-children turn out to be. I'm not sure I gave them much of a choice, but they didn't fight it either. Perhaps they were wise enough to understand that allowing me to chase what I thought was my dream would show me what a good thing I had left behind.

I had convinced a friend from Harvard to go with me. We first flew down to Martinique and then made our way over to Antigua. We pitched a tent up on a hill overlooking a place called English Harbor. It was beautiful. Every morning, we would go down to the dock to see if anybody needed a couple of crew members. Three long weeks went by without any takers, but we persisted and eventually landed a job as deckhands on an 83-foot Bermuda Ketch named *Isabell* that had been scuttled during World War II to keep her away from the Germans.

My friend went back to the states after a couple of months, but I was determined to stay the course. I was paid next to nothing, something like $1.50 an hour, but I did have free room and board. My sleeping quarters were in the fo'c'sle, in the front of the boat where it comes to a point at the bow. If I woke up in the middle of the night with a dream, I would hit my head on the underside of the deck, which was only about six inches away. But it was fantastic. I didn't sail around the world, but I worked on *Isabell* for a year, rising to first mate and sailing from one beautiful Caribbean island to the next. The boat was chartered by paying guests, most of whom were American, while all the other crew members were British. It was hard work at times but mostly fun to be with beautiful people on a beautiful yacht in beautiful places where the trade winds almost always blew. And it also was enlightening because I realized that hedonistic living had its limitations and—seeing its effects on those who had adopted it as their main goal—I began to understand the value of an education.

Returning to Harvard, I found a new and very small major called "visual and environmental studies," which was kind of their concession to the creative arts. It wasn't art history, which would've been much more their style, so they made it very small. Only about fifteen students per class were admitted, and I was fortunate to be one of them. I took a fascinating mix of classes, from filmmaking and photography to architecture and city planning. I didn't inherit any of my father's artistic talent, but I gravitated toward creative endeavors and eventually decided that I wanted to move toward a career in media.

And it would be media that eventually led me to healthcare. After graduating from Harvard in 1974, I got a job with IBM, not selling computers but as an intern in their corporate communications department. While working on their corporate advertising campaign, I met a filmmaker who hooked me up with a venture capital funded company called Playback Associates, which was an early producer of home video programming. Playback was acquired by a public company called Reeves Communications, which was a major producer of network sitcoms and made-for-TV movies. So, I had achieved my goal of landing in the media industry, but somehow, I still didn't feel fulfilled.

While I was at Reeves, however, I found a passion producing health-related television programming and ultimately left to start a company called American Medical Communications (AMC) so that I could concentrate in this area, as it corresponded with a lifelong personal interest in health and fitness. After that, I launched the first cable TV channel devoted exclusively to health, America's Health Network (AHN), which we eventually sold to FOX when it became clear that the internet was filling the need I had designed AHN and AMC to fill—to give consumers easy access to reliable health information.

After the sale to FOX, I had to figure out what to do next. I experimented with consulting for a while but kept coming back to my passion for healthcare. One of the things I had noticed at AHN was that viewers who were calling in to our "Ask the Doctor" programs frequently said they were doing it because they either didn't have a primary care physician or couldn't make a timely appointment if they did. This started me thinking about how I could help to fill this need—to make high-quality, basic healthcare more accessible and affordable. This became my true passion and my focus during the next twenty-plus years.

The purpose of this book is to share with you my experience in helping to "retailize" the healthcare industry. We often take it for granted that there's a walk-in clinic nearby, but basic healthcare has become significantly more accessible today than it was when I began my quest to make it so. When I started down this path, in 2001, it was impossible to get a vaccination, medical test, or prescription anywhere other than at a doctor's office and only by appointment—if you could get one.

Today, millions of people benefit every day from accessible, affordable healthcare at walk-in clinics close to their homes that are open seven days a week with extended weekday hours, providing high-quality basic healthcare at reasonable prices that are transparently posted. During the recent pandemic, the entirety of the United States benefited from the access to COVID-19 testing and vaccinations that these clinics provided. It is notable that, over the last five years, the use of retail-based clinics has grown 200 percent and urgent care clinics 70 percent, while emergency room usage declined by 1 percent, and claims filed by primary care practices declined 13 percent.

But these retail clinics did not emerge without a fight, as they faced strong opposition from the medical establishment, overly restrictive government regulations, and skeptical third-party payors, not to mention consumers who were conditioned to believe that quality healthcare could only be delivered in an office or a hospital on someone else's schedule and without having any idea of its cost.

This is not to diminish the importance of physicians and large health systems, which continue to play indispensable roles in patient care, but the fact is that the huge healthcare system that has been built on this foundation has not proven to be accessible or affordable enough for many patients and third-party payors. The system needed to be disrupted, and I am proud to be one of a relatively small number of people (including many of my teammates) who were able to do it.

However, this is not a book about unbridled success, as many "business books" are. It is the story of how things really go when you are crazy enough to try to effect significant change in a multi-trillion-dollar industry. The fact that retail-based and urgent care clinics are now a permanent part of the healthcare landscape is evidence of some success, but getting to this point has been a wild and, frequently, very rough ride that challenged all the passion, endurance, and street smarts I could muster at every step along the way.

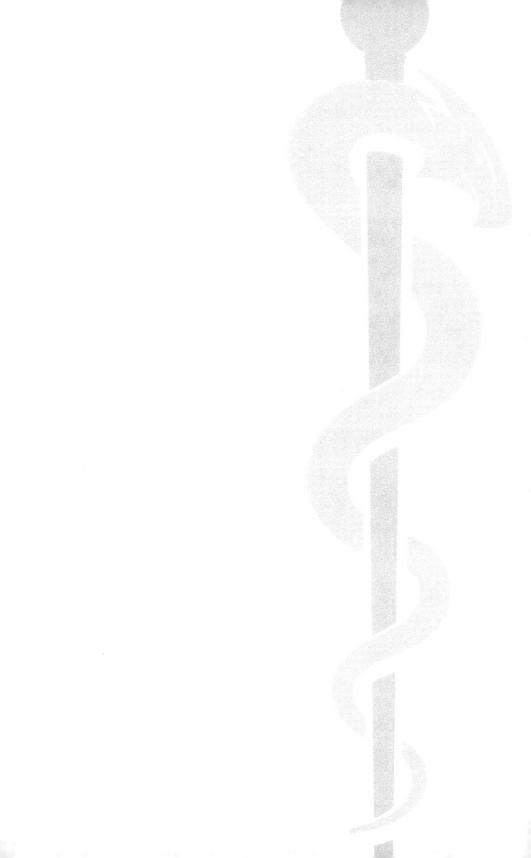

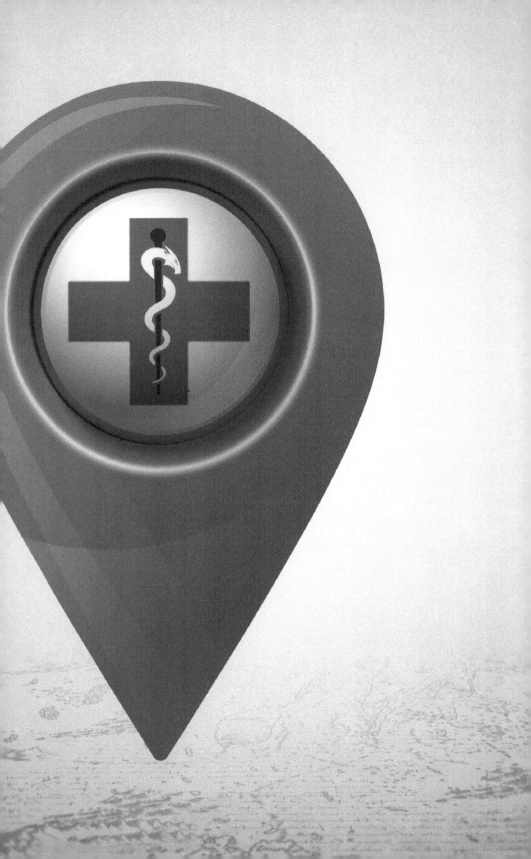

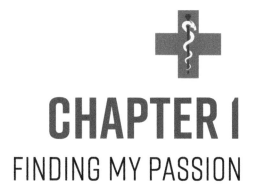

CHAPTER I

FINDING MY PASSION

I didn't start thinking seriously about life after college until the last semester of my senior year at Harvard. I remember going over to the Office of Graduate and Career Plans to see which companies were still interviewing, and the only one where I could see any connection with what I thought I wanted to do was IBM. At the time, IBM was leading the computer revolution, and they were doing a lot of corporate advertising and sponsoring specials on network television as part of a campaign to convince opinion leaders that they were Big Blue, not Big Brother. With my interest in media, and my major in visual and environmental studies, I thought there might be an opportunity for me to work on their campaign.

The man I interviewed with wanted to turn me into a computer salesman, but I had no interest in that. I told him that I was interested in doing media work at IBM, and so he put me in touch with their vice president of corporate communications. I interviewed with him and a few others in his department, and they offered me an internship. This was when IBM was being sued by the U.S. Justice Department for being "cold, monopolistic and predatory" because they had about 85 percent of the computer market. Part of IBM's response was to burnish their image, and, in a rather naïve way, they decided they needed to infuse some young blood into their corporate communications programs to help them connect with the counterculturally oriented baby boomer generation. So, they created an internship program at their corporate headquarters in Armonk, New York, and hired five people including me who were straight out of college.

I really had no idea what I was doing or what the job might entail, but I still remember that first day at IBM, going down to the corporate dining room. Literally, everybody there except me was wearing a dark suit, a white shirt, a tie, and lace-up black shoes. I wasn't wearing any of those things and didn't have any of them in my closet. I was coming right from Harvard's radicalized campus of 1974, where long hair, headbands, and tie-dye T-shirts were the norm. It was a bit of a shock, both to them and to me.

But I found it interesting because IBM allowed me to work on their sponsored TV specials and exhibitions, corporate advertising, and several internal communications projects. One of them was an annual IBM event where the company gave "Outstanding Invention" and "Outstanding Contribution" awards. The invention awards were given to employees who had developed technologies that might have been worth many millions of dollars, and while the recipients received fairly large checks for their good work, the amounts were probably nothing compared to the commercial value of their patents.

The outstanding contribution awards went to employees who had accomplished meaningful things on the business side of the company. I was particularly impressed with one that was given to a manager who had killed a very large project he was leading because he felt that it wasn't going anywhere and would end up costing the company a lot more money for no real benefit. I thought this was a very enlightened decision on the part of both the manager and the company. I ended up being the project manager of a book profiling all the award winners that year, which was fascinating because I got to travel all over the country to interview the award winners.

When I arrived at IBM's offices in Northern California where many of their engineers worked, I saw that the atmosphere was nothing like the headquarters in Armonk. Gone were the dark suits and ties. In were tennis sneakers and open-collar shirts. The engineers I interviewed had beautiful offices nestled in the hills of what subsequently became known as Silicon Valley. They could come and go as they pleased, and they didn't look or act anything like the prototypical IBMer. It was clear that IBM had figured out that to attract and retain the kind of engineering talent they needed to keep the company on the leading edge of information technology, they had to dispense with the straight jacket and be more flexible.

Toward the end of my two-year internship, in 1976, I was assigned to work on a bicentennial exhibition sponsored by IBM at the Kennedy Center in Washington, DC, celebrating two hundred years of the performing arts in America. It was a fantastic experience, as I was working with some of the most talented exhibit designers in the world to bring an endlessly fascinating subject to life for millions of citizens who were able to attend the exhibition free of charge due to IBM's sponsorship. At the end of my internship, IBM offered me a permanent position. It was tempting, but despite the amazing experience I had at IBM, I just couldn't see myself as a lifer in a large corporation.

I also worked on some of IBM's corporate advertising during my internship and, along the way, met a talented documentary filmmaker named Greg Shuker who was shooting commercials for IBM's ad agency, Geer DuBois. I was assigned to go on location as IBM's representative when they filmed some of these commercials, and over time, Greg and I became friends. I eventually shared with him that while I was enjoying my internship at IBM, I wasn't going to stay with the company and was looking for something in the media business. He was kind enough to introduce me to some friends he had at a new company called Playback Associates that was backed by a leading venture capital firm called Venrock (started with Rockefeller family money) that was trying to capitalize on the developing market for home video programming, and they offered me a job.

The challenge for Playback was that not enough consumers had VCRs yet, so the consumer market for original programming was too small to build a business around. Realizing this, the company pivoted to the corporate market where large companies were beginning to use videos for management communications and training. This wasn't exactly the kind of programming I had hoped to produce, but it gave me valuable experience and many lifelong friendships.

One of my best friends at Playback was John Bunyan. He was very smart (had gone to Stanford), was about my age, and actually lived in our office at 30 Rockefeller Center because they weren't paying either of us enough to be able to rent most apartments in Manhattan (I was still living in my mother's rent-controlled apartment, which she had vacated). One day when we were presenting to a big corporate client in our office, I needed to get a writing utensil so I could take notes. John's desk was close by, so I casually opened the right-hand drawer and out popped his dirty laundry. I don't think we got that piece of business, but we certainly got a lot of laughs out of it.

It was also interesting to work for a venture-backed company. This was in the very early days of venture capital, and Playback was in Venrock's portfolio along with Apple Computer and Eastern Airlines. I hadn't known anything about venture capital, so it was a revelation to discover that there were firms that specialized in providing capital to early-stage companies. That exposure to the world of venture capital would come in handy later.

Playback was producing programming for many large companies, including Union Carbide, Johnson & Johnson, and Phillips Petroleum. It was interesting work with good people, but it wasn't creatively challenging (lots of talking heads), and it became somewhat repetitive, so I was open to a change when I was approached by IBM's ad agency, Geer DuBois, about going to work for them. I was more interested in television programming than in advertising, but Geer DuBois was a very creative agency, so I decided to give it a shot. Predictably, they assigned me to work on the IBM account, which was their biggest client, and eventually also on the Insurance Company of North America (INA), their second-largest account, which later evolved into Cigna.

After a couple of years at Geer DuBois, I was promoted to vice president and account supervisor and was making good money, but I wasn't passionate about the work. I was just kind of going with the flow and having perhaps too much fun as a bachelor in New York City. And then Playback approached me about coming back because they were starting to expand. Playback had just been acquired by Reeves Communications Corporation, a large, publicly traded entertainment company best known for its production of network television series including *That's Incredible!*, *Gimme a Break*, and the Emmy Award–

winning *Kate & Allie*. They also had a very successful division in Los Angeles that produced made-for-TV movies and production facilities in New York City that included the iconic Ed Sullivan Theater. I was attracted to the opportunity because it seemed closer to what I wanted to do, and I felt like the opportunity at Playback would be bigger with Reeves behind it.

Playback was one of several companies Reeves had acquired to provide various kinds of communication services to corporate clients and their ad agencies, including production of video programming, creation of audio-visual support for client sales and management meetings, and supplying video production and editing facilities. I returned to Playback as a vice president and was promoted to president when my friend John Bunyan departed for another opportunity. Later, when all five of Reeves' corporate services entities were combined into one unit, I became president of the Reeves Corporate Services division. This was a huge challenge because I hadn't been running Playback for very long and thus had very little experience running one company, let alone the much larger and more diverse division that resulted from the merger of multiple companies. Needless to say, I was in way over my head!

Each of the merged companies had their own president, all of whom were considerably older than I was. They had not been enthusiastic about being folded into a single division or reporting to someone they viewed as inexperienced, so I had to learn how to manage people without being overly directive. My strategy for getting them to cooperate was to convince them that I was there to support them, which worked quite well and was my first experience with what is commonly known today as "servant leadership"—though I had not heard the term or read anything about the philosophy at the time.

Perhaps the best part about running Reeves Corporate Services was meeting my future wife, Allison. She was running retail marketing for EF Hutton, a leading stock brokerage firm at that time. They had developed an advertising campaign with the tagline, "When EF Hutton talks, people listen." It became one of the most iconic advertising campaigns of all time. As one blogger wrote recently, "There is no doubt that EF Hutton was responsible for one of the most recognizable and memorable ad campaigns of the 1970s and '80s."[6]

My former boss at Geer DuBois, Fred Irwin, introduced me to Allison. Geer DuBois was doing some advertising for EF Hutton, and she had asked Fred if they would also produce video programs for management development and marketing, but they were not interested. In those days, many advertising agencies just did advertising and shied away from other forms of communication, which didn't make sense to me because I think companies should use all available channels in a consistent manner to maximize the cost-effectiveness of their internal and external communications. In any case, Fred introduced Allison to me, knowing that Playback was one of the few companies with a significant track record in corporate video programming.

I met with Allison and pitched her on our capabilities and eventually won the business. I began working on the EF Hutton account personally because it was a big piece of business. We were producing a lot of programs for them, including programs that were used to educate their brokers on new financial products. I remember one particularly ambitious program about an innovative new investment vehicle that allowed EF Hutton's retail customers to make a single investment that would give them ownership in all the companies that

---

6   SF School of Copywriting blog, "Great Ad Campaigns: 'When EF Hutton Talks,'" April 4, 2022, accessed July 17, 2023, https://www.sanfranciscoschoolofcopywriting.com/great-ad-campaigns-when-ef-hutton-talks/.

were created when AT&T was broken up. To make a long story short, Allison and I developed a personal relationship outside of business (which she claims began over a dinner she had scheduled to tell me that she was firing us), and eventually we married in 1985.

While I continued to focus on building Reeves Corporate Services, I was also given the title of senior vice president of Reeves Entertainment Group and vice president of the parent company. I began working on sitcoms including *Kate & Allie*, which was creatively challenging and fun, but I wasn't passionate about what I was doing. I just didn't feel like I was contributing to society in any fundamental way.

Around this time, I was introduced to a couple of individuals who had a thriving business called TransMedica that specialized in creating continuing medical education (CME) programs for physicians that were sponsored by pharmaceutical companies. To maintain their licenses, physicians have to earn a certain number of CME credits every year, which at that time they mostly did by attending pharmaceutical company–sponsored conferences usually held in vacation resorts. While these conferences were fun for physicians, they were not a very efficient way to provide education, and they were increasingly coming under scrutiny by regulators who questioned the objectivity of the information that was presented (which tended to support the use of sponsors' prescription drug products) and the ethics of providing physicians with what were essentially free vacations.

As an alternative to this traditional approach, TransMedica came up with the idea of producing and airing regularly scheduled televised programs that would keep physicians and other healthcare professionals up to date on the latest developments in medical science and clinical care. These programs would be sponsored by the same pharmaceutical companies that were sponsoring CME conferences, but they would have no editorial input, and physicians could get their CME credits in the comfort of their own homes.

TransMedica proceeded to buy airtime in early morning slots on network affiliates and independent stations throughout the country, and Reeves Corporate Services—with me as executive producer—began producing regular weekly series with consumer-unfriendly names like *Cardiology Today* and *Morning Rounds* in an ad hoc network that was called MD/TV. Pharmaceutical companies had never advertised their prescription drugs on TV before, but they were intrigued by the idea. One of the main obstacles was that they didn't have any commercials, so we had to produce those, too.

> I BEGAN TO SEE THAT CONSUMERS HAD A THIRST FOR RELIABLE HEALTH INFORMATION. THAT WAS THE BEGINNING OF WORKING ON SOMETHING I WAS REALLY PASSION-ATE ABOUT—WHERE I FELT I WAS FILLING A REAL, UNMET NEED.

As we started to get viewership data from around the country, I noticed that while the programs had a predictably high concentration of physician viewers, the majority of viewers were consumers. This was not surprising because the only health-related information generally available to consumers at that time was through short segments on the evening news or a handful of sports-specific publications, and it confirmed my suspicion—as a health, sports, and fitness nut—that consumers had a thirst for reliable health information that was not being quenched. Why else would they get up at 5:30 in the morning to watch programs designed for board-certified internists? More importantly, that was the beginning of working on something I was really passionate about and where I felt I was filling a real, unmet need. It was an opportunity to do well by doing good, as they say.

I was so excited about the concept that I pitched Reeves' senior management on making a big commitment to health and medical programming for consumers. Health was a universal concern, I told them, and my experience with MD/TV suggested that viewers would be even more responsive if the health content was designed to be understood by them and presented in a way that was consistent with commercial television production values. Their response was that I should forget about this serious health and medical stuff and focus on taking advantage of the new opportunities they had given me in the Reeves Entertainment Group. But I had finally found my passion, and nothing was going to stop me from following through on it.

In the course of producing the MD/TV programs, I had met a talented, Houston-based cardiologist named Vincent Friedewald. He was the host of *Cardiology Today*, and we had helped to turn him into one of the first "TV docs." As we got to know each other better, Vince and I started talking about building on a small production company he had started called American Medical Video to create a much larger one solely dedicated to the production and distribution of health-related programs for professionals and consumers, which was more or less the same idea that Reeves had passed on. Vince then introduced me to one of his patients, Ted Gaylord, who was a very successful businessman. Ted was also based in Houston, but he came to New York on business frequently, and I got to know him well enough that Vince and I eventually told him about our idea for the new company, and he offered to provide the seed capital for it.

That was 1988. Alison and I had just had our first child in New York City, Joseph Webster "Jeb" Golinkin II, named after my father, and we were thinking of moving out of the city anyway. Both Vince and Ted were based in Houston and had strong connections at the Texas Medical Center, one of the world's largest medical centers. This was a nice coincidence, as Allison was originally from Texas. She had grown up in the Rio Grande Valley and moved to Austin with her parents when she was in high school. Later, she graduated from the University of Texas in Austin, and in 1988, her parents and siblings were still living there. So, from a business and personal perspective, it made sense to move to Houston. We packed up and headed west.

Allison continued working for EF Hutton up until the time we made the move. She had been promoted to senior vice president, making her one of the most senior women at the company, and she had recently been featured in a *New York Times Magazine* article about the new cadre of female executives on Wall Street. But like my mother a generation before, she had her own stories about the challenges of being a successful woman in a male-dominated workplace. Because of her job title, she was permitted to eat in the executive dining room, but she rarely did because it was clear that many of her male colleagues frowned on her being there. Her response to this subtle discrimination was to tell the CEO that he didn't have to worry because she didn't want to eat with them either.

My mother was living alone in New York City after my father's death, and she hated to see us go, but she had been career-oriented herself and was very supportive of anything I wanted to do, no matter how crazy it seemed. So, I moved to Houston and lived in a residential hotel alone for a couple of months, while Allison and I tried to find a house before she and Jeb moved down permanently.

This was just after the economic crash in Houston, which had busted after the oil boom of the late 1970s and early 1980s. We had sold our two-bedroom co-op in New York City and hoped to be able to trade it for a house big enough for a young family. I was hopeful in this regard because housing prices in Houston had tumbled more than 30 percent over the previous few years, but we had to make it work because Allison had resigned from EF Hutton and I had a new job with a young company that didn't pay much and wasn't very stable.

We found a good real estate agent who showed us a number of attractive houses. There was one we particularly liked, so we arranged to see it for a second time with Allison not knowing how much it was likely going to cost. At the end of the showing, we met with the owner, and I asked him how much he would take for his house if we paid cash. He hesitated for a minute and then gave us a price that was considerably less than what we had sold our much smaller apartment in New York City for. I breathed a sigh of relief, but Allison couldn't contain herself. "Is that all?" she asked. Not the greatest negotiating tactic, but we quickly made a joke out of it and lived happily in that house for many years.

Vince (as chairman) and I (as CEO) named our new company American Medical Communications (AMC), and we rented offices in a three-story townhouse in a transitional neighborhood in Houston called Montrose. Today, it's very trendy and hip, but it certainly wasn't back then. I think we rented the entire townhouse for less than $1,000 a month. The dining room was our conference room, and the upstairs bedrooms were our offices. It wasn't fancy, but we were in business.

With Ted's capital, Vince's on-air personality and connections, and a talented producer named Donald Goodwin who I had become good friends with at Playback, we began producing health-related TV programs and series that were sponsored by pharmaceutical and other health-related companies. We had multiple series running on Lifetime and the Discovery Channel. In addition to the televised programming, we acquired a small company called Infotronics that produced video programs for ophthalmologists, OB-GYNs, and other physicians to educate their patients about upcoming procedures and to document informed consent. Traditionally, doctors had provided this education in person, but our programs freed them from this repetitive but critical task. The programs helped ensure that everything a patient needed to know was covered in a standardized way: what the procedure involved, how to prepare for it, what to expect afterward, and the risks and potential complications.

In order to fund our growth, we needed to raise more capital than Ted was willing to provide, so we hired a local investment banker, prepared a presentation and private placement memorandum, and hit the road. I had never raised money for a company before, so this was all new to me, and I had no idea how much time- and energy-consuming it would be. I ended up making more than sixty investor presentations to raise about $2 million from venture funds in Houston and Boston, so we were successful in the end, but it was a long, hard struggle. It was frustrating to have to spend so much time and energy raising money that I could have spent building the business, but I knew that we would not be able to grow without it. I also found that the feedback we received from presenting AMC's business plan to sophisticated investors could be used to refine the plan in important ways, as long as I listened carefully even though I was mostly selling.

One day not long after we completed the capital raise, I was listening to the radio while driving and tuned into a program called *Ask the Doctor*. The format basically revolved around a local physician taking calls from listeners, and it had become quite popular. I thought it made sense because it was simple to produce, and the doctor was being responsive to what consumers wanted to know rather than him deciding what he thought they should know.

I thought there was potential in expanding this concept to television where some of the answers to viewers' call-in questions could be visualized (remember that this was still in pre-internet days). Pursuing this idea, we produced a pilot and ran it on a local TV station. We used the same doctor I had heard on the radio program as our host, and while he wasn't made for prime-time television, I could see how it could work with different talent and production values.

The *Ask the Doctor* pilot was a wake-up call for me. All my observations and experiences suggested that there was a significant consumer demand for easier access to reliable health information presented in an understandable and entertaining manner, and yet there was no single place consumers could go to find it. Even with all of AMC's programs, consumers had to hunt around for them. *What if we went bigger and bolder?* I thought to myself. *Why not start a twenty-four-hour cable TV network devoted to health?* There were successful subject-specific channels—such as CNN for news, MTV for music, or ESPN for sports—but there was no channel devoted to health. In addition, the "Ask the Doctor" format could provide an inexpensive programming foundation for just such a channel.

Once again, many of my colleagues, friends, and probably even family thought I was crazy. I knew that AMC would not want to pursue this. The capital needed to start a twenty-four-hour cable channel was well beyond the company's means, and Vince seemed happy doing what the company was doing. I went to AMC's investors and told them that I understood why they wouldn't want to take the company in this direction but that I wanted to pursue it and would give them my equity in AMC in return for the company waiving all rights to the *Ask the Doctor* pilot and the concept behind it.

Meanwhile, my wife, Allison, was busy raising our two children (George Willeford "Will" Golinkin, named after Allison's father, had been born in 1990), and I was now out of a job. But I believed strongly in this new vision, so I retreated to the small home office Allison had set up for me in our garage to write a business plan for what would become America's Health Network (AHN).

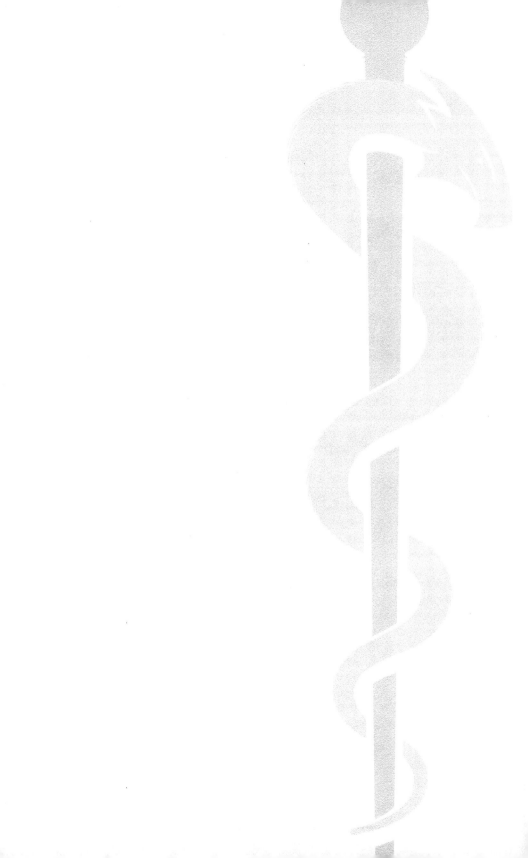

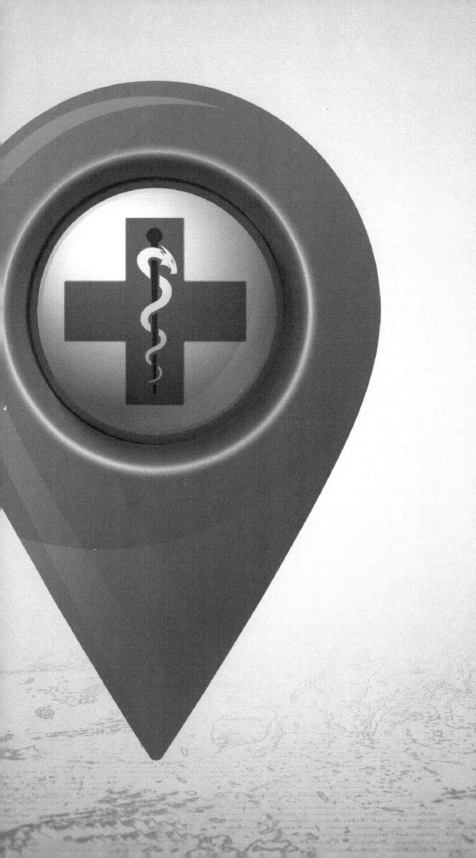

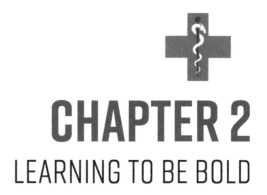

CHAPTER 2
LEARNING TO BE BOLD

As the business plan for America's Health Network (AHN) began to take shape, I realized that I needed to find a great partner to help bring my vision to life. By this point in my career, I had a lot of experience in the development, production, and distribution of health-related programming, but starting a cable TV network from scratch was a whole new ball game. I needed a partner who had experience in this area and who was more operationally oriented than I would have the time to be.

I knew just the right person. I had met Joe Maddox years earlier when I was working at Geer DuBois and he was selling advertising for *The Wall Street Journal.* He had gone on to become an early executive at the Discovery Channel and had joined me briefly at American Medical Communications (AMC). I shared my plan for AHN, and fortunately he was interested. Together we started to put some meat on its bones with the understanding that I would be the CEO and he would be the COO.

There were several formidable challenges to launching a cable TV network in the early 1990s, including one that was somewhat unique to a health channel. We needed content, and a lot of it, to fill up twenty-four hours a day, seven days a week of airtime. However, there wasn't much health-related programming available for us to license (for all the reasons previously mentioned), so we would have to produce most of the programming ourselves.

I thought we could leverage the "Ask the Doctor" format into multiple series, each of which would be devoted to a particular specialty that would draw significant viewership: primary care, pediatrics, OB-GYN, cardiology, sports medicine, and so forth. The programs in these series would be relatively inexpensive to produce, but their success would depend upon our ability to recruit knowledgeable physician hosts with compelling on-camera personalities, make the programs visually interesting, and secure a large facility with multiple sound stages for their production.

Joe was based in Orlando, Florida, and had some connections with the local theme parks. Nickelodeon, the cable TV channel for kids, had built a large production facility on the perimeter of Universal Studios Florida that enabled theme park visitors to tour the studio and serve as audiences for their live programs. (My son, Jeb, was later "slimed" on one of these programs and still refers to it as one of the highlights of his childhood.) We decided to try to replicate that model and, after many meetings with universal executives, convinced them to let us build our studio next to Nickelodeon's. The catch was that we didn't yet have the money to do this, but we thought that having the agreement would help us raise it.

We also needed a highly credible medical content partner that would—among other things—help to assure the cable TV operators we were trying to convince to carry AHN that the health and medical information being disseminated would be evidence based and not drag them into malpractice suits. In this regard, as well, launching a health network was uniquely challenging. But once again, fate smiled upon us.

In the process of looking for potential investors, a friend introduced me to his contact at Allen & Company, a highly regarded boutique investment bank in New York City that specializes in media and entertainment deals. Allen & Co. thought the AHN plan had potential, so they, in turn, introduced me to executives at a small but growing, Minneapolis-based company called IVI Publishing, which had recently acquired the electronic publishing rights to the *Mayo Clinic Family Health Book*, then considered the bible of consumer-oriented health information.

The only problem with the book—then in its second edition—was that it had grown to more than 1,400 pages, so it was not easy for consumers to find the answers they were looking for. IVI solved this by putting the book's content on searchable videodiscs, and they were enjoying considerable success with this electronic version. IVI saw our new cable health network as a logical extension of their strategy to expand in health-related electronic media, so they ultimately decided to invest $2 million in AHN in conjunction with a commitment to help secure Mayo Clinic as AHN's medical content partner.

Mayo turned out to be a wonderful partner. They saw AHN as a vehicle to promote their brand nationally and to extend their involvement in electronic media even beyond their partnership with IVI. My main editorial contact at Mayo was Dr. David Larson, editor of the *Mayo Clinic Family Health Book*. He was a senior physician at

Mayo who had originated the idea of publishing a medical reference book for consumers. David worked with other senior physicians at Mayo to create the content for the book, with each one writing a section related to their specialty. David then edited all these drafts for accuracy, stylistic consistency, and readability. I was in awe of the breadth and depth of his medical knowledge and his commitment to excellence. It was a pleasure and an honor to work with him and with Mayo generally. I have collaborated with many well-established health systems over the years, but if I ever have a serious health problem, Mayo will be one of the first places I turn to for care.

Another challenge of the cable business in the early 1990s was that while viewership was growing, ratings were still low compared to broadcast network programs. As a result, there was not a lot of advertising revenue flowing to cable TV channels. To compensate for this, we decided to sell AHN-branded products on air. We would source the products ourselves and make sure they were relevant to each of our "Ask the Doctor" programs. For example, we would sell pacifier thermometers during our "Ask the Pediatrician" segments. We ultimately hired an executive with experience sourcing these types of products and negotiating private label deals with manufacturers. Also, Allen & Company introduced us to Barry Diller, the former president of ABC and then controlling shareholder of the Home Shopping Network (HSN). As a result, HSN agreed to provide customer service and fulfillment for our branded products.

Another challenge of starting a cable channel in the early 1990s— perhaps the most daunting—was getting cable operators to carry AHN on their basic tier, hopefully without charging exorbitant "carriage fees." Joe and I knew we needed an experienced salesperson who could lead this effort, and again we were fortunate to attract Bruce Sellers as our EVP of affiliate sales. Bruce was an industry veteran who had held this position at QVC and other well-established cable TV channels. We also added other key team members in the process of assembling an impressive management team.

But more than anything else, we needed to raise a large amount of capital to implement our plan. With the limited funds we had raised from IVI, we had assembled a top team and inked partnerships with Universal Studios Florida, Mayo Clinic, and the HSN. Still, we were quickly running through these funds, and IVI was not in a position to provide additional funding.

We hired Allen & Company as our investment banker, and they introduced us to the Providence Journal Company, which owned the *Providence Journal*, the largest newspaper in Rhode Island, along with several other newspapers. They also owned broadcast TV stations, operated cable systems in multiple markets, and had just made their first investment in cable programming with the Food Network. The Providence Journal Company liked our plan for AHN, and after multiple meetings with their executives, they asked me to present to their board of directors at an upcoming meeting.

I flew to Providence for the presentation, expecting to be on their agenda near the beginning of what was supposed to be a morning meeting. I was not only excited about the opportunity to present but also nervous because we were running out of money, and I knew that the Providence Journal Company was exactly the kind of strategic investor we needed to get AHN off the ground and maximize its chance of success. As it turned out, the board had multiple emergency matters to discuss, and my presentation was repeatedly delayed. Meanwhile, I nervously twiddled my thumbs, waiting to go on stage. At about 5:30 in the afternoon, they finally called me in. After telling their board at the beginning that I had "peaked" after waiting more than eight hours, I made my presentation, and they apologetically but enthusiastically approved the investment.

At the closing dinner in June 1996, I cited a quote from Goethe that my experience has repeatedly proven to be true: There is one elementary truth, the ignorance of which kills countless ideas and splendid plans: the moment one definitely commits oneself, then Providence moves too. All sorts of things occur that help one that never otherwise would have occurred. ... Whatever you can do, Or dream you can do, Begin it. Boldness has genius, power and magic to it. Begin it now.

We were off and running. We built a 16,500-square-foot production facility at Universal Studios Florida, hired sixteen physician hosts, and developed a system for enabling them to visualize their answers to viewers' call-in questions using a Telestrator, similar to what John Madden was then using to diagram plays during NFL games. The device allowed our hosts to electronically "draw" on digitized medical images from the Mayo Clinic and other sources that were stored in our library and served up on demand.

While our programming was well received and our viewership was growing, it was still a challenge to get our network on many cable systems. Bruce Sellers was doing his best, and I was accompanying him on many cable operator presentations, but it was slow going because there were hundreds of operators in markets throughout the country that had local decision-making authority even if they were owned by larger companies. In addition, AHN was the last independent basic cable TV channel to be launched, and we were up against programming behemoths like FOX and ESPN. They had multiple networks and could get new ones carried by threatening to remove their already popular channels that cable operators depended upon. These programming conglomerates also used their leverage to extract "subscription fees" from cable operators. For us, it was the opposite: we usually had to pay fees to the cable companies to get AHN on the air.

We did get a couple of big breaks. Early on, Cablevision picked us up in the New York metropolitan area, the largest cable market in the country. Then we were picked up by DirecTV, which gave us national coverage. That was back when DirecTV subscribers had to install huge satellite dishes in their backyards to receive the programming. We referred to them as "bird baths," and I had one installed in my backyard in Houston. The local cable operator, Time Warner Cable, was still not carrying AHN, so I needed to get DirectTV just to watch our own channel. Still, DirectTV was growing rapidly, providing some competition to local cable TV monopolies. Also, we were gaining carriage in other markets and starting to secure some high-profile advertisers, including many of the pharmaceutical companies I had worked with at AMC.

We also launched AHN.com as the internet companion to our cable network. This was when the internet was taking off, and we received international publicity when we broadcast the first live human birth on the internet. We followed this up with the first live, open-heart surgery, performed by the famous heart surgeon, Dr. Denton Cooley. Certainly, we were burning cash—as all cable networks do at the beginning—but we were on budget and moving forward as planned. Until one day, when it all changed.

In 1997, our majority investor, the Providence Journal Company, was acquired by A.H. Belo Corporation, which owned *the Dallas Morning News* and other major market newspapers. A.H. Belo also owned broadcast TV stations around the country, but they had no presence or experience in cable TV. It quickly became apparent that they did not want to be in the cable TV programming business, and particularly with AHN because we were still burning cash. I met with their CEO shortly after the announcement of the acquisition, and he told me that they were no longer going to support AHN and that we needed to find a new investor or a buyer. I told him that, in this case, they should return their controlling stake to us so that we would have something to sell to a new investor, and he agreed.

All of this was very depressing, but we were rapidly running out of cash, so I had no choice but to get back on my proverbial horse and try to find a new investor or buyer. I had been talking to some of the large healthcare systems for some time about airing our programs in their hospitals, which would have grown our viewership and been very appealing to health-related advertisers. This naturally led me to Columbia/HCA, which was the largest for-profit hospital chain in the country. Somehow, my idea made its way up to Rick Scott, who was then the CEO of Columbia/HCA. Scott later became the governor of Florida and currently serves as a U.S. senator.

Rick liked the concept. He is a very smart and aggressive executive, and he saw an opportunity to use AHN to promote the Columbia/HCA brand nationally. He also understood the advantages of airing our network in Columbia/HCA hospitals and, ultimately, made an offer to buy the whole company. After multiple rounds of negotiation, we agreed on the price and terms, and all the documents were prepared for closing. But literally on the day we were scheduled to close, news broke that Columbia/HCA was being investigated by the federal government for Medicare fraud. Rick was ousted, and the deal was off. It was a very dark day with a bittersweet end, as I arrived back in Houston to find that Allison and my great friend, John Beckworth, had met me at the airport to celebrate the closing they presumed to have occurred.

At that point, we were totally out of cash. I mean, we were running on fumes, so Joe and I had no choice but to furlough 90 percent (more than two hundred) of the company's employees. The only good news was that because we had produced a huge amount of relatively timeless original programming over the past couple of years, we were able to keep the network on the air by rebroadcasting old shows.

While keeping AHN on the air with a skeleton crew, I madly scrambled to find an investor that could put us back in business. A friend in New York put me in touch with Howard Millstein, a major real estate developer in New York City. He thought AHN had potential and agreed to extend us a bridge loan, structured as a convertible note. In other words, if we could not pay back the loan, he could convert it into equity and control the company. Companies in dire financial straits often have to resort to these kinds of deals, which are often referred to as "loan to own" arrangements.

But then we caught a break when Rick Scott came back into the picture, saying he wanted to make a personal investment in the company. While Columbia/HCA was in big trouble and would ultimately plead guilty to fourteen felonies and pay a massive fine to the U.S. government, Scott had not been charged. He bought a controlling interest in AHN, and we used some of the proceeds to pay off the loan from Milstein.

Rick was supportive in many ways, but he was new to the cable TV business. Also, his involvement was a mixed blessing in our efforts to gain carriage on cable systems because there was a lingering threat that he would be indicted (which he never was). There were some people who thought Rick was brilliant and had just gotten a raw deal, while others were wary of getting involved due to the legal cloud that hung over him. It was a challenging situation, so we decided that, if we had the opportunity, it would probably be best to sell AHN.

At the time, there was one other cable TV network devoted to health, FitTV, though it was more focused on fitness as its name suggests. Jake Steinfeld, a fitness guru and colorful character, was the driving force behind it. FOX had invested in FitTV, so I thought the media giant might be interested in AHN, as well.

I was introduced to Pyper Davis, a bright and able executive who had worked for Rupert Murdoch at News Corporation (owner of FOX and many other media assets) and was running FitTV. She and I both thought there might be an opportunity to merge the two networks. Health and fitness on one channel would make filling up the airtime easier and would expand the appeal of both networks. Also, FitTV and AHN had geographically complimentary subscriber bases, so the business combination made sense on multiple levels. Pyper and her team (including the president of FOX Networks Group) invited Rick and me to San Diego to watch the San Diego Padres and the New York Yankees play in the 1998 World Series. At the game, we reached a verbal agreement to sell AHN to FOX.

I stuck around for a couple of months after the sale, but I could see AHN/FitTV was going to have trouble getting the support it needed to grow. The combined network had landed in FOX's sports programming group, and it was apparent that their management team was totally focused on their regional sports networks and didn't really understand or care about health and fitness. Their view seemed to be that FOX's senior management had decided to acquire AHN so they were going to play along, but it clearly wasn't a priority.

After trying unsuccessfully to get FOX's sports programming management to share my vision for the combined network, I decided to exit rather than be party to what I viewed as the inevitable dismantling and ultimate decline of something that had been so near and dear to me—and which, more importantly, I believed was serving a real need. Two years later, in 2001, FOX sold AHN/FitTV to the Discovery Channel, and it eventually was folded into Discovery Health. But the FOX connection had certainly helped with distribution. At the time of the sale to Discovery, the combined subscriber base was more than twenty million.

With AHN behind me, I had to figure out what to do next. I had been renting an apartment in Orlando and traveling constantly during my time at AHN, so I was looking for something a little easier where I could spend more time with my family. A friend of mine, Frank Krasovec (who had introduced me to Allen & Company), approached me about becoming chief marketing officer (eventually also vice chairman) of a company he was running called Norwood Promotional Products. His offer was appealing because I liked and respected Frank, Norwood was a market leader, and it was based in Austin, not too far from Houston, so I would be closer to home.

Norwood was a large company with about $600 million in annual revenue and divisions all over the country that put corporate logos on different kinds of products, from baseball caps and polo shirts to golf balls and Koozies. It was a good gig and challenging in its own way, but as had happened early in my career, I didn't feel like I was contributing much to society. It just wasn't for me, so I started looking for something more meaningful.

I wrote a business plan for a Spanish language website called "Salud America" because I could see that the Spanish-speaking population in the United States was growing rapidly and had the same need for access to reliable health information that everyone else did. I made a deal with Rodale Publishing, which was then the leading publisher of health and fitness magazines, to license the Spanish language rights to their content. I even got two billionaires interested in investing in the new venture, Mike Milken, the junk bond king, and Carlos Slim, the Mexican mobile phone tycoon.

What I remember from visiting Mike and Carlos at their respective compounds in Los Angeles and Mexico City is that they were very intelligent and that their security was intense. I still recall being picked up at the Los Angeles Airport by one of Mike's drivers in a heavily armored suburban who told me in response to my questions about his background that he had previously been a Los Angeles Police Department (LAPD) precinct captain. For a number of probably fortuitous reasons, the business never got off the ground, but it was a memorable chapter nevertheless.

IN MY HEAD, THE SAME QUESTION JUST KEPT COMING BACK TO ME: HOW CAN I HELP THESE PEOPLE, AND OTHERS LIKE THEM, GET EASIER ACCESS TO HIGH-QUALITY, AFFORDABLE HEALTHCARE?

Throughout this diversion, I kept coming back to an idea that had occurred to me at AHN. We had thousands of viewers calling into our "Ask the Doctor" programs, and many of their questions started the same way. They would begin by expressing how thankful they were to be able to ask the physician host a question because either they didn't have a personal physician or they couldn't get in to see them on a timely basis. In my head, the same question just kept coming back to me: *How can I help these people, and others like them, get easier access to high-quality, affordable healthcare?*

Trying to answer that simple question became a passion that has consumed all my professional attention for the past two decades.

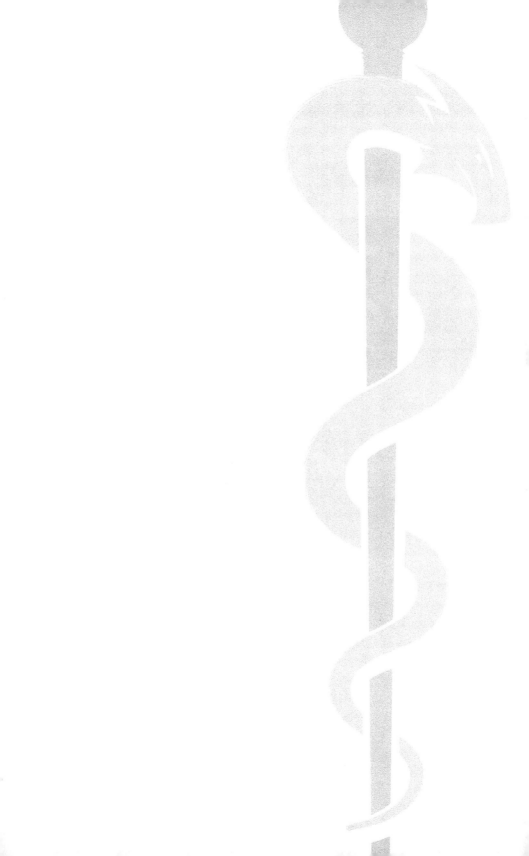

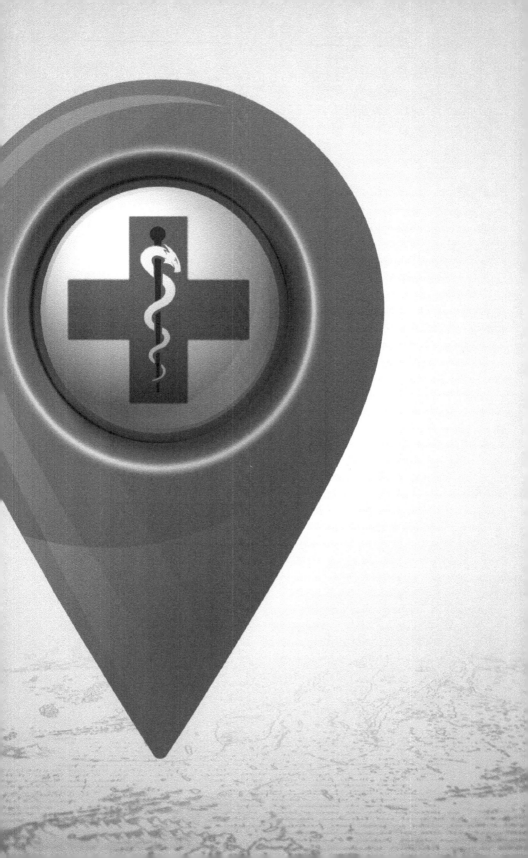

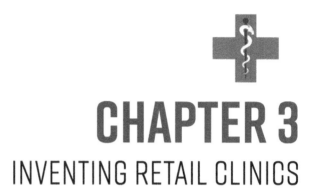

CHAPTER 3
INVENTING RETAIL CLINICS

With the goal of building a business around giving consumers easier access to high-quality, affordable healthcare, I started trying to figure out how I was going to achieve it. In early 2001, Walt Mischer, a good friend and very capable healthcare executive and entrepreneur, told me that he had invested in InterFit Health, a start-up that was staging health screening events in Randall's grocery stores in Houston.

I visited a few of their events and saw that what they were doing had potential. They were setting up tables near the in-store pharmacies and administering basic screenings (blood pressure, cholesterol, osteoporosis, etc.), as well as more sophisticated medical tests that required blood draws. The blood samples would then be sent off to a lab with the results reported on a password-protected website. InterFit also administered flu shots in the fall. I could see that there was demand for these services, and I thought that the business could be expanded to other retailers and possibly include a broader range of services.

I shared my impressions with Walt, and he ultimately asked me to join InterFit as their CEO. We began to expand the screening events in Randall's stores. When Randall's was acquired by Safeway, it gave us the opportunity to expand in their stores nationally. We also started doing screenings for Albertsons nationally and ultimately landed a contract with Walmart to do screenings and flu shots in their Supercenters, including a few events where we administered flu shots to shoppers in all their roughly 2,500 Supercenters on the same day.

These monster events were exciting, but they almost killed the company because we had to hire thousands of temporary employees all over the country, relying on them to administer the screenings, tests, and immunizations properly and to accurately and honestly collect payment from hundreds of thousands of customers. We eventually addressed the payment issues by working with Walmart and one of their marketing agencies, North Star, to secure sponsors for the events, which made them free to customers, but it was clear that continuing to scale the business would be a logistical nightmare.

However, one of the things I kept hearing from our customers was that while they valued the access to our screenings, tests, and immunizations, they wanted us to expand our range of services. Reflecting on this, I concluded that the only way we could expand in a meaningful way would be to put permanent locations in the stores. This would also help solve another problem: customers had a hard time finding our events because we only conducted them on certain days and in specific stores. If we had permanent locations, finding us would be easy.

Now I felt like we were onto something. *What if we opened small medical clinics inside retail outlets?* We could focus on drugstores, grocery stores, and big box retailers that had already invested in healthcare through their pharmacies. And we could treat patients with a limited set of acute/episodic conditions and provide the kinds of basic preventive care we had been offering at our screening events.

The value proposition for patients was compelling. The clinics would be located inside nearby retail outlets. They would be open seven days a week with extended weekday hours, just as their host retailers were. Patients could get in and out quickly because we would treat only a limited set of common conditions that could be managed in about fifteen minutes each—such as colds and flu, ear and urinary tract infections, and minor abrasions. In addition to the preventive services we had been offering on an event basis, we could also offer other commonly needed health-care services, such as school and sports physicals and drug tests.

Even if there was a line at these walk-in clinics, patients would at least know how long it would be because visit durations would be predictable. Plus, they could shop in the host stores while waiting for us to call their cell phone or text them when our provider was ready to see them. In addition, if we wrote them a prescription, they could walk across the aisle to get it filled at the in-store pharmacy rather than having to make a separate trip.

The value proposition for host retailers was equally compelling. The clinics would attract patients to their stores, many of whom would patronize their pharmacies and purchase other products while they were waiting. In addition, host retailers could increase productivity and reduce health benefit costs by encouraging their employees to use the less expensive in-store clinics rather than going off-site when they needed basic care.

As I envisioned it, these clinics would also reduce health-care costs for both patients and third-party payors because we would staff them with less expensive Advanced Practice Providers (APPs)—nurse practitioners and physician assistants—rather than physicians. In general, APPs are masters prepared in their respective specialties, and research had shown conclusively that they were more than capable of providing care that was comparable in quality to physician care, if not even better, within the limited scope of services our clinics would be offering.

Sounds great, right? Patients, retailers, and payors all win. Win-win-win. What's not to like? The answer was almost everything if you were an integral part of the healthcare delivery and health insurance system that predominated at the time.

The first thing I had to do was to find a good name for InterFit's new business. InterFit would continue as the "events-based" business, but we thought we needed a new name for the in-store clinics. By that time, I had become aware of another company that basically had the same idea. It was called Minute Clinic, and their tagline was "You're Sick, We're Quick." While I believed that convenience and speed would be an important driver of success, I felt that their name and tagline were slightly off in terms of overemphasizing just one aspect of the value proposition in a business where quality was critical. Working with North Star, we eventually landed on the name RediClinic.

Next, we needed to determine the optimal size of our in-store medical clinics. Eventually, we settled on about 500 square feet, with at least two exam rooms and a fully functional restroom. Minute Clinics, by contrast, turned out to be smaller, usually with only one exam room, and relied on their host stores' restrooms. As a result, they were less expensive to build than RediClinics.

However, I thought our additional capacity would be important for several reasons. First, having more space would help us attract and retain APPs and ancillary staff members. Who wants to be stuck in a cramped room all day? Second, having more than one exam room would greatly increase patient volume and productivity. While one patient was being prepared by our medical assistant in one exam room, our APP could be treating a patient in another one. In addition, having a restroom would increase both the perception and reality of quality. As it was, Minute Clinic patients needing a drug test would have to pee in the store's restroom and then walk back across the store with their urine sample in hand!

The next order of business after rebranding the company and settling on a design concept was to convince retailers to give us some space in their stores so that we could test the concept. This was not easy because it was a new and unproven idea, and retailers were notoriously focused on revenue per square foot as the key determinant of what products or services to offer in their stores. Since I had no idea how or where RediClinics would be successful, we decided it made sense to test them in several different venues: drugstores, grocery stores, and big box retailers. Each had different advantages. Big box retailers had the highest foot traffic and thus the most potential customers. Drugstores had far fewer shoppers, but they had the most logical connection in consumers' minds with healthcare services. Grocery stores with pharmacies were somewhere in between.

We started with the largest grocery chain in Texas, H-E-B, because we had done some screening events in their stores, and they were in my backyard. H-E-B was also the largest private employer in the state with more than 80,000 employees. I knew that employee healthcare costs were an issue for H-E-B, so I thought they might be interested in how in-store medical clinics could reduce these costs while generating incremental sales. Fortunately, they were interested and agreed to lease space to us in a store in Tomball, Texas, a suburb of Houston.

Walmart was a bigger challenge. The people we had worked with on the screening events had moved on to other positions, and the person at Walmart who was responsible for leasing space at the front of their stores to third parties (banks, cell phone stores, nail salons, etc.) thought my idea was crazy.

However, after many meetings, he finally relented and offered us space in a couple Walmart stores that had vacancies, which usually meant that the stores were not very successful. The two stores he offered us were in out-of-the-way towns in Oklahoma: Broken Arrow and Owasso. Pretending not to be very excited (I would have taken anything), I told him rather boldly that I would sign the leases for the two stores in Oklahoma but only if he would agree to give us space in one of the Supercenters near their corporate headquarters in Bentonville, Arkansas.

Miraculously, a few weeks later, he called back to say that space had opened up in a store in nearby Fayetteville, Arkansas. I snapped it up without even asking about the terms of the lease because I figured it would be helpful to be in a location where Walmart executives and their family members could personally experience how great (I hoped) our service would be.

Now, we had secured pilot spaces in both grocery stores and big box retailers. All we needed was a drugstore. Also, while we had committed to lease space in rural and suburban settings, I thought it would be good to try RediClinic in an urban one.

Donald Goodwin, who I had worked with at both Playback and AMC, introduced me to mid-level executives at Duane Reade, the largest drugstore chain in New York City. After a few meetings with them, I made my way up the chain to Duane Reade's CEO, Anthony Cuti. Tony was a character (later sentenced to prison for securities fraud) and drove a hard bargain in the classic New York manner—take it or leave it! He liked the idea and had space in one of their stores just north of Times Square, although only on its second floor. At the time, Duane Reade had one of the highest sales per square foot of any retailer in the city, and he wouldn't give us the space unless we could match their current productivity. At something like $85 per square foot (about $3,500 per month), I knew it would be tough to make the economics work, but I gulped hard and agreed to the deal. I thought that having a New York City location would help us raise money, which we desperately needed to open clinics in the spaces we had already leased.

Meanwhile, InterFit was still doing reasonably well, but it was a small business and was not generating the kind of cash that could have supported the growth of RediClinic. Therefore, we needed to raise a significant amount of money from an institutional investor. Donald came through again and introduced me to some people who were working closely with Steve Case, the founder of AOL. After famously selling AOL to Time Warner in 2000, Steve had used some of the proceeds to form a new investment firm, called Revolution Health, with the goal of revolutionizing the healthcare business. As in the case of Duane Reade, I eventually made my way up the chain and was able to schedule a meeting with Steve and a few of his closest associates at Revolution's offices in Washington, DC.

The presentation was on a Friday afternoon, and the meeting seemed to be going well. However, it was taking longer than I expected, and I needed to catch a flight back to Houston. My younger son, Will, was playing in a tennis tournament that weekend, and I had promised to take him. I had missed too many of my sons' events when I was at AHN and was not about to miss this one. But here I was meeting with the founder of AOL! Still, I excused myself, grabbed a cab, and barely made my flight. I got back to Houston, picked up Will at home, and started the long drive to Corpus Christi where his tournament was to be played. Along the way, I was thinking that maybe I had blown the deal of my life by leaving the meeting with Steve Case early. Just then, I got a call from one of Steve's associates. They wanted to make a large investment in RediClinic.

It took one more presentation in Washington, DC, to finalize the deal to Revolution's board—which included General Colin Powell, Netscape founder Jim Barksdale, Hewlett Packard CEO Carly Fiorina, and other luminaries. It seemed to go well, and I remember being particularly heartened when General Powell gave me a "thumbs up" as Walt and I were leaving the room. They agreed to the investment, and we were ready to launch.

We opened RediClinics in all five of the leased spaces we had secured and anxiously awaited the results. The initial feedback from patients was extremely positive. They were blown away by the convenience and relatively low cost of the care we provided. However, there was one major problem: we didn't take insurance. Our cash prices (initially $49 per visit) were lower than all other providers, but they weren't lower than the $20 co-pays that insured patients usually paid when they went to a doctor or the "free" care (paid for by taxpayers at a much higher cost than $49) that many uninsured patients received if they sought care at an emergency room. The inevitable conclusion was that we would need to get contracts with all the major health insurers to survive.

The problem was that large health insurers including United, Aetna, Humana, and Cigna were reluctant to contract with Redi-Clinic for several reasons. One, it was a new and unproven concept. A medical clinic in a grocery store? Two, we used APPs to deliver the care instead of physicians, which made third-party payors question the quality of our care. And three, they were getting pressured by the physicians in their provider networks and the medical societies that represented them to avoid doing business with us because they thought we threatened the viability of their practices by being more accessible, affordable, and transparent with our prices, which were posted in the check-in areas for all patients to see.

This was the beginning of the war against RediClinic and other retail clinic providers by the medical establishment, whose strategy was to claim that we could not possibly be providing quality care delivered by APPs in drug, grocery, and big box stores.

I was convinced that the quality of our care at our clinics was at least comparable to that provided by other healthcare providers—within our limited scope of practice—but I knew we needed a credible third party to validate this. Fortunately, the Rand Corporation, a well-respected research organization, stepped up to the plate and performed a comprehensive study that compared the quality of care at Minute Clinics to that provided at physician practices, physician-staffed urgent care clinics, and emergency rooms. What they found was that the quality of basic care at the Minute Clinics was comparable, if not slightly better, than that provided in the other delivery outlets.[7]

The publication of these research findings marked a turning point in the development of RediClinic and other retail clinics, as it gave third-party payors, including Medicare and Medicaid, the air cover they needed to meet the needs of their members by contracting with us. That should have been game over, but it wasn't because there were numerous state regulations that had been advocated by physician lobbying groups that prevented RediClinic from being able to fully deliver on its value proposition.

In Texas, for example, there was a regulation that every APP had to enter into a collaborative practice agreement with a local physician who had to be available 24/7 and actually be on site during 20 percent of the hours that the APP was providing care. The result was that we had to pay physicians to provide this oversight even though they were not providing care, and in our case mostly either sitting around doing emails or buying groceries in one of our H-E-B host stores. And this was all happening in a state that had and still has a severe physician shortage.

In response to this, I contacted the Texas Medical Association (TMA) and told them that if they didn't relax the physician on-site requirement and expand the number of APPs a single physician could collaborate with (which was a maximum of three at the time), I would take my case to the media and describe these regulations as an unconscionable misallocation of physician resources. Ultimately, the TMA gave way in stages, first reducing the on-site requirement

---

7   Robin M. Weinick, et al, "Policy Implications of the Use of Retail Clinics," Rand Corpo-
     ration, 2010, https://www.rand.org/pubs/technical_reports/TR810.html.

to 10 percent and then eliminating it entirely, but it took them two years to do it.

In New York, we faced other kinds of regulatory challenges. I suspect that with generous political support and strong advocacy from the State Medical Society of New York, a regulation had been enacted that prohibited the "corporate practice of medicine." While this kind of regulation—which also had been enacted in other states—was intended to prevent for-profit companies from being able to influence the type and extent of medical care provided to patients, the result of it was that every healthcare clinic or practice in New York State had to be owned by a physician. This was problematic for RediClinic because we relied on APPs to provide the care in our clinics but needed to find physicians to agree to own these professional corporations even though they weren't practicing in them.

In addition, we had to go through the expensive process of setting up management companies to provide services to these physician-owned professional corporations as the only way of making our clinics financially viable. Furthermore, regulations had been enacted in New York that prohibited providers from advertising the comparative cost of their services, which was one of our main selling points as the lowest-cost provider. I did my best in meetings with regulators and the Medical Society of the state of New York (read physician lobbying group) to convince them to make exceptions in our case so that we could provide New York residents with easier access to high-quality, affordable healthcare, but they refused to give in. Eventually, this forced us to exit the state because the legal costs of dealing with the prohibition against the corporate practice of medicine and fighting the ban on comparative advertising were too heavy to bear.

I pointed all of these out in an editorial published in the *The Wall Street Journal* in August 2007, titled "Health Care When You Want

It." In the editorial, I acknowledged that some physician-backed medical organizations had by then seen the light about retail-based clinics and, if not supporting them enthusiastically, were at least not aggressively opposing them like the American Medical Association (AMA) and some state and specialty-specific physician organizations. Before submitting my editorial to the paper, I sent a draft to Steve Case and Ron Klain, who was then serving as Revolution's general counsel (subsequently as President Biden's Chief of Staff). Ron wanted me to soften the statements I was making about the opposition we were facing from the medical establishment, but—to his credit—Steve overruled him.

> I LIVED IN CONSTANT FEAR THAT A SINGLE, WELL-PUBLICIZED MISTAKE IN DIAGNOSIS AND TREATMENT AT ONE OF OUR GROWING NUMBER OF CLINICS, OR AT THE GROWING NUMBER OF COPYCAT CLINICS THAT WERE CROPPING UP ALL OVER THE COUNTRY, COULD DERAIL THE ENTIRE INDUSTRY.

While the Rand study was an important tool in putting the quality issue to bed, I lived in constant fear that a single, well-publicized mistake in diagnosis and treatment at one of our growing number of clinics, or at the growing number of copycat clinics that were cropping up all over the country, could derail the entire industry. In order to address this threat, in 2006, I supported Hal Rosenbluth, the founder and CEO of a competitor retail clinic operator called "Take Care," in creating the Convenient Care Association (CCA). Its charter was to advocate for member retail clinic operators, provide clinical and management support to their employees, and ensure that member organizations were meeting CCA's minimum quality standards. Membership in CCA grew to include companies and health systems representing more than 90 percent of all retail clinics nationally and achieved its goal of helping to assure that quality care was being provided. In the process of helping to start the CCA and ultimately serving as its president for five years, I learned a tremendous amount from my competitors and developed lifelong friendships with many of their leaders.

In just three years, we had opened RediClinics in the stores of some of the nation's leading retailers—to the delight of hundreds of thousands of satisfied patients—raised growth capital from one of the biggest names of the internet era who was now bent on revolutionizing healthcare, contracted with all of the nation's largest health insurers, survived stiff opposition from the medical establishment, and even begun to effect much-needed federal and state regulatory changes.

But there was one critical challenge remaining: turning Redi-Clinic into a profitable business.

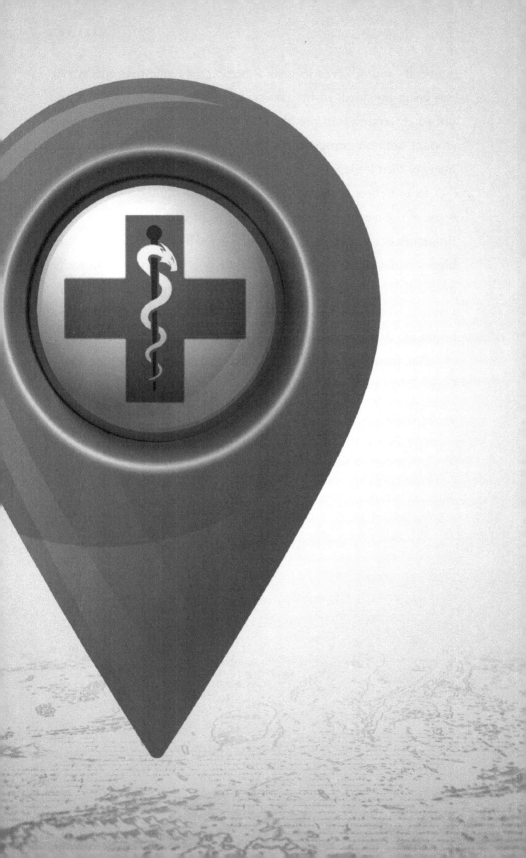

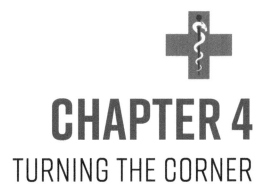

CHAPTER 4
TURNING THE CORNER

With Revolution's money behind us, RediClinic was expanding rapidly with all three of our retail partners in the original markets as well as new ones in Texas and Arkansas and, subsequently, with Walgreens in Atlanta. While it was exciting to be on a fast growth track, I wasn't comfortable that we had a scalable model, and the financial results reflected this. Individual clinic profitability was uneven, and with the additional cost of a rapidly growing corporate overhead, we were burning cash at an alarming rate. But this was the way Revolution seemed to want it—consistent with their dot-com heritage and its emphasis on growth at the expense of profitability—so I felt like we didn't have much of a choice.

The crux of the problem was that we didn't have the right management team in place to create the unit economic model and be able to scale RediClinic in a profitable manner. We had exited the retail screening and flu shot business so that we could concentrate solely on RediClinic, which obviously had much greater potential, and had changed the name of the parent company to RediClinic. However, in many cases, we were still relying on early InterFit employees who—in some cases—had difficulty adapting to a new business model that was much more sophisticated and challenging.

While relying on InterFit teammates to make the adjustment to RediClinic wasn't working particularly well, Revolution's approach to building our management bench didn't work much better. Shortly after Revolution had made their investment, they pushed me to engage the executive search firm, Spencer Stuart, to help us find an operationally oriented president with multi-unit retail experience. After interviewing multiple candidates, I narrowed the search down to two individuals who I thought had the most potential. One had been an executive at Blockbuster, and the other had run Chase's retail operations. I was concerned that neither had any healthcare experience and that both were more accustomed to operating in much larger companies with far more resources. Still, both candidates had deep operating experience, so I passed them on to Revolution for their feedback. The next day I got a call from one of Revolution's board members, Frank Raines, the former CEO of Fannie Mae and budget director in the Clinton administration. He said they wanted me to hire both of them!

I didn't think hiring two people for the same job was going to work out well, and I should have pushed back harder, but Revolution was trying to be helpful, and I knew we needed a deeper bench. As it turned out, it didn't work for some of the reasons I had feared, mainly a lack of healthcare experience and a big-company mentality. Also, they were essentially competing with each other from the start, and if the truth be told, they probably wanted my job as well. Neither of the executives lasted much more than a year, leaving us essentially back to square one from a management standpoint.

The challenge of putting a team together for RediClinic was compounded by the fact that it was hard to find senior-level executives who had both multi-unit retail and healthcare experience and who also had an entrepreneurial bent. We had proven that traditional multi-unit retail experience was not enough, largely because there were important nuances to the healthcare business that confounded most retail veterans. Most importantly, they had to learn that it was difficult to compete on price alone because a large portion of the cost of care was paid by third parties. Also, there were a myriad of regulations and operational concerns that were specific to providing healthcare services, some of which were linked to patient morbidity and even mortality. On the other hand, recruiting the right talent from within the healthcare industry was also challenging because many of the largest providers at that time were nonprofits with limited consumer marketing experience and entrepreneurial savvy.

Fortunately, I ran into just the right person and in the nick of time. Danielle Barrera came to RediClinic via Memorial Hermann Health System, then the largest health system in Houston. My partner, Walt Mischer, had been on the board of Memorial Hermann and served as their interim CEO for a couple years. It had always been my conviction that RediClinic should not stand apart from the traditional healthcare ecosystem but should instead be integrated into it for the benefit of our patients, many of whom came to us with conditions that were outside of our limited scope of practice and needed higher levels of care.

Partnering with health systems made sense from that perspective because it would help to ensure "continuity of care," and I also felt that the affiliation with a well-known health system would lend credibility to our new company. This would help to attract not only patients but also the providers we were trying to recruit and the third-party payors we wanted to contract with. Health systems would benefit from a partnership with RediClinic, as well, because we could push their brands out into their communities in ways it was otherwise difficult and expensive for big hospitals to do, and they would also benefit from our downstream referrals.

Despite these apparent benefits, most health systems at that time wanted nothing to do with us because we were new and unproven and because we were seen as threatening to many of their affiliated physicians. In part due to Walt's high-level contacts, however, Memorial Hermann was an important early exception, and they agreed to enter into an exclusive, co-branded partnership with RediClinic in Houston.

Danielle was a mid-level executive who wore many hats at Memorial Hermann and had been assigned to manage their partnership with RediClinic. We got along well from the start. I could see that she was very competent and operationally oriented. I also could see that while she had been at Memorial Hermann for more than ten years, she had an entrepreneurial spirit that was looking for an outlet. Others at RediClinic were equally impressed, so we eventually offered her a job as vice president of operations. It was a pretty risky bet for her to leave the comfort and security of a multi-billion-dollar, not-for-profit health system for the insecurity of an early-stage company that was competing in a new sector of the healthcare industry. I suspected that she took some comfort in the fact that we were backed by Steve Case and Revolution Health, but little did Danielle and I know at the time that this and many other things were about to change.

The first shoe to drop was that we lost our partnership with Walgreens. Less than a year earlier, Walgreens had agreed to host

RediClinics in more than twenty of their Atlanta stores, and things seemed to be going very well. However, in May 2007, the large drugstore chain suddenly announced that they were acquiring one of our competitors, Take Care. Prior to this announcement, Walgreens executives had told us that they were pleased with our partnership and with the performance of our clinics in their stores. They also indicated that they were interested in exploring the possibility of acquiring us. However, the terms they initially proposed were tough, and Revolution wasn't interested in selling. Losing Walgreens was very disappointing, but I believed we could make it without them as long as we had Revolution Health behind us and were continuing to partner with other large retailers.

A year earlier, in 2006, CVS had acquired Minute Clinic, so the new reality was that our two largest competitors—Minute Clinic and Take Care—were now owned by the two largest drugstore chains in the United States, CVS and Walgreens. This eliminated two of our most logical investors or acquirors. As a result of Walgreens' decision, Danielle's very first job was to close all our Atlanta clinics and transfer them to Take Care. I figured that anyone who could survive this initial experience and still want to keep going was tough enough to survive anything, as she turned out to be.

The next big shoe to drop was Steve Case's decision to start winding down Revolution Health. He had started the bold venture capital firm with a big bang and hired a lot of very smart but expensive people. However, healthcare was proving to be more difficult to revolutionize than I guess he thought it would be, and I certainly could relate to that. Nevertheless, it was a big blow to us because we were still burning cash and had been counting on Revolution to fund these early losses. But Steve had made up his mind, and he was quite generous in selling his controlling stake back to the existing shareholders at a discount from what Revolution had paid for it.

The final, almost nail in the coffin was something we could not have anticipated. In classic Walmart style, after we had essentially proven out the retail clinic concept in a small number of their stores, they decided that they wanted to aggressively expand and invited nearly all the retail clinic companies in the United States—irrespective of size and experience—to compete in a "bake off" for a much larger contract. We were invited to participate, but now we had to beat out more than thirty companies that were vying for the opportunity to open potentially hundreds of clinics in Walmart stores. It was frustrating to be in that position after all the work we had put into educating Walmart on the business, but we threw ourselves into the bake off—which was more like a shark tank—and ultimately won the competition.

After several rounds of negotiation, we emerged from the process with a contract to open an initial one hundred RediClinics in Walmart stores in markets to be determined. This was a huge victory for us, but at this point Revolution was out of the picture, so we would have to raise a considerable amount of money from entirely new investors to open and sustain these clinics to cash flow breakeven. However, with the Walmart contract in hand, we were confident we could do it.

In mid-2008, we hired Credit Suisse as our investment banker and went to work creating the presentation and private placement memorandum with the goal of raising tens of millions of dollars at an aggressive valuation. More as a courtesy than anything else, our banker first introduced us to the merchant bank within Credit Suisse that invested the bank's own money alongside their clients' money in private equity deals. They loved our presentation and wanted to invest practically on the spot, but we felt like we might be leaving money on the table by taking an offer from the first prospect we had solicited, so we told them that we greatly appreciated their interest but needed a few weeks to consider other offers.

What we didn't anticipate is that literally the following week, in September 2008, the global financial crisis and the subsequent "Great Recession" formally began with the bankruptcy of Lehman Brothers. All financial markets locked up, effectively eliminating the possibility that we would be able to raise equity capital at a valuation that wouldn't crush our existing shareholders. We even went back to Credit Suisse's merchant bank with hat in hand, but they told us that they now wouldn't be able to invest at all. The result was that we had to inform Walmart that we didn't have the capital to support the contract. They reacted by pulling the plug on the roughly twenty RediClinics that we were already operating in their stores.

At that point, we had already pulled out of Duane Reade stores because of the regulatory challenges of operating in New York. We had also lost our Walgreens clinics due to their acquisition of Take Care, and we were now in the process of closing down our Walmart clinics—and doing it during the worst financial crisis since 1929.

Our prospects looked bleak, but I still believed in RediClinic, and we still had H-E-B as a partner in Texas, which was one of the few parts of the country where the economy was still growing. Walt and I felt that we had a chance to save the business if we retrenched and focused on finally creating a profitable clinic model that could be scaled in the future when the economy improved.

We had our work cut out for us, but it was easier to concentrate on refining our business model when we had thirty clinics in our Texas backyard that were located inside the stores of a retailer who valued the services we were providing than it had been when we had one hundred clinics spread all over the country and were playing whack-a-mole every day. By then, Danielle had been promoted to chief operating officer, so we rolled up our sleeves and started to dig in.

The economics of the retail clinic business were relatively simple. RediClinic was a high fixed cost business, with labor (APPs and ancillary staff members) being by far the largest component. With our average net revenue per patient, which was largely determined by third-party payor contracts, we needed about twenty patients per day to break even at the clinic level. More than thirty patients per day produced significant profits, but less than twenty produced equally significant losses. Therefore, having a consistently high volume of patients was essential to the profitability of our now much smaller company. It was clear to me from publicly available information that most Minute Clinic and Take Care clinics were not profitable on a stand-alone basis, but they didn't need to be because they contributed to the profitability of their owners' drugstores. We couldn't afford that luxury.

A number of key factors impacted our ability to achieve consistently high patient volumes at our clinics, some of which were common to all multi-unit retail businesses while others were unique to our provision of healthcare services. In the former category, we needed to make sure our clinics were located in areas that predisposed them to be successful. As RediClinic's business had grown, we were able to collect more data on our patients and used this data in deidentified form to refine a statistical model that was able to predict with reasonable accuracy whether a clinic would be successful if located in a particular area.

In general, we found that the most successful locations for Redi-Clinics were in middle-income areas with many dual-income families with children in their homes. The healthcare decision-makers in these homes (predominantly women) were pressed for time and thus embraced the convenience we offered. Another general finding was that we did better in high-growth areas that attracted new residents who usually didn't have established primary care relationships. With that said, we generally found that more than 40 percent of our patients said they didn't have a primary care provider, which is one of the reasons our nation's healthcare system is so costly (more on this later). We had to close some locations in Texas that had been opened early on without the benefit of our new site selection model, but we also opened new ones that were successful partially because of it.

> **WE GENERALLY FOUND THAT MORE THAN 40 PERCENT OF OUR PATIENTS SAID THEY DIDN'T HAVE A PRIMARY CARE PROVIDER, WHICH IS ONE OF THE REASONS OUR NATION'S HEALTHCARE SYSTEM IS SO COSTLY.**

Assuming our clinics were located in high-potential areas, we found that the two biggest drivers of patient volume were satisfied patients telling their family members and friends (#1) and shoppers who saw us when they visited our host stores for other reasons (#2). With respect to the latter, our success was always tied to the size of our host stores' foot traffic to some degree, but generating high levels of patient satisfaction was largely within our control, and we attacked that with a vengeance.

Since it had been clear from the beginning that patient satisfaction was largely determined by the attitudes and capabilities of our patient-facing team members (never "employees"), we decided to build our entire organization around attracting, training, motivating, and supporting those team members.

In order to attract and retain the best patient-facing team members, we knew we had to create a culture that was driven by a sense of mission, which we defined as "to provide consumers with easy access to high-quality, affordable healthcare." We also needed to define our core values and insist upon honoring them. In addition, we needed to ensure that patient-facing team members felt supported in our clinics, which could get very hectic at times with as few as three team members handling more than thirty patients per day.

Our philosophy was that our patient-facing team members should never feel that all management cared about was the money, even though we understood all too well that there was no mission without the profits to support it. Team members had to believe that we in the corporate office, which we referred to as "Support Services," were there to support them and not the other way around. I have always believed in what has been called "Servant Leadership," and our executive team took every opportunity to display it.

The result of our relentless focus on both patient and team member satisfaction was very high customer service ratings. Like many other companies, we used a measurement of customer satisfaction called a "Net Promoter Score" (NPS), which asks a single survey question: "On a scale of 0 to 10, how likely is it that you would recommend our organization to a friend or colleague?" Based on their responses, customers (in our case, patients) are categorized as Promoters, Passives, or Detractors, and then the percentage of Detractors is subtracted from the percentage of Promoters to calculate the organization's NPS.

RediClinic's NPS was consistently higher than 85, which was unheard of in healthcare or any other industry. To ensure that it stayed that way, we bonused patient-facing team members based on their clinic's Net Promoter Scores, which was the one thing they could control and what we believed was the most important ingredient for current and future success.

While patient satisfaction and our in-store presence were always the best means of attracting new patients, advertising and other forms of promotion also played a role. While we had little success with traditional forms of media, such as newspaper ads, direct mail, or billboards, we had more success with newer forms of advertising, including paid search and search engine optimization (SEO), which means optimizing how you appear in Google search results. When consumers had a health issue, they were increasingly turning to the internet and their smartphones for guidance, so we tried hard within our limited means to make sure RediClinic showed up as an option and that patient reviews supported a decision to choose us.

Our growing number of affiliations with large health systems helped to attract new patients as well. Building on our early experience with Memorial Hermann in Houston, we developed co-branding partnerships with other leading health systems, including Methodist in San Antonio and Seton in Austin.

In addition to leveraging the awareness and credibility of their brands, RediClinic benefited from these partnerships in other ways. Health systems were often one of the largest employers in their local markets, and their employees became frequent users of our in-store clinics. We also received referrals from their affiliated physicians, who felt less threatened than before because we had systematically assured them that we would not steal their patients but would actually help to strengthen their patient relationships by providing them with after-hours, weekend, and overflow care.

In the case of Seton, and later with other large health systems, we entered into formal joint ventures, where the health system either purchased a stake in our existing clinics in their market or agreed to invest alongside us in new markets. This enabled us to expand in a capital-efficient manner. We might not have had a multi-billion-dollar drugstore chain behind us, but we were committed, creative, and nimble.

While strong patient volume was the key to financial success, we had to make sure we were getting accurately paid for the care we provided to the large percentage of our patients who were covered by health insurance plans. There were two main parts to this challenge.

WE MIGHT NOT HAVE HAD A MULTI-BILLION-DOLLAR DRUGSTORE CHAIN BEHIND US, BUT WE WERE COMMITTED, CREATIVE, AND NIMBLE.

The first part was to ensure that our patient-facing team members collected the right amounts from our insured patients at the time of service. This was not as easy for us as it is for a typical physician practice where patients usually make appointments in advance, thus giving the practice time to figure out what plan the patient is on, whether their deductible has been met, and what co-pay or co-insurance amount should be collected. In our case, since most of our patients were walk-ins, our "Patient Service Advocates" had to figure all this out on the fly and in the context of trying to deliver on our promise of a fifteen-minute visit.

The second part of the payment challenge was that we had to make sure we were properly reimbursed by the health plans for the balance of the cost of each visit, which became an increasingly challenging problem as we were now accepting literally hundreds of insurance plans (be careful what you wish for!). This required a much more sophisticated electronic medical record system than the crude "RediRecord" system we had developed internally when we launched in 2004. Therefore, in 2008, we converted to Athena, then a new system that helped us reduce our bad debt.

It had been a rough few years. Our main investor had backed out, our partnerships with three of our four original retail chains had been terminated, our two main competitors had been acquired by huge companies that were investing heavily in their growth, and the nation's economic woes made it impossible to raise growth capital from financial sources. Nevertheless, we were still alive and kicking in the great state of Texas and slowly but surely turning RediClinic into a real business.

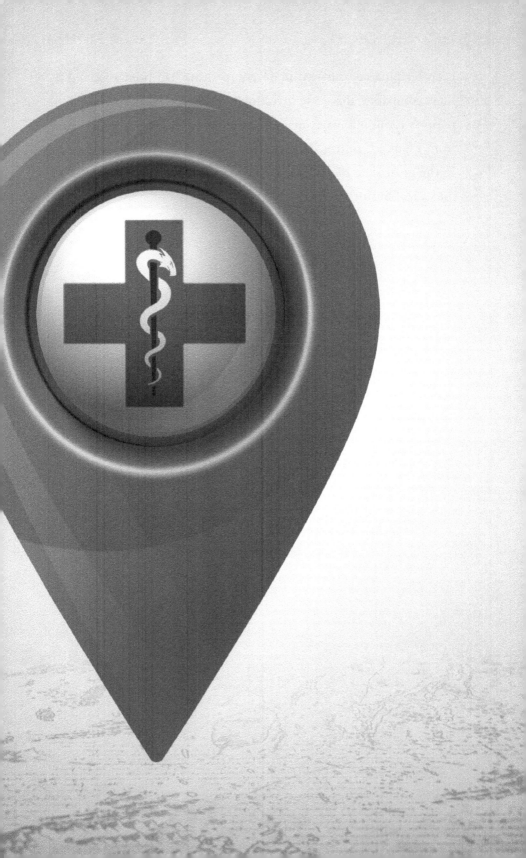

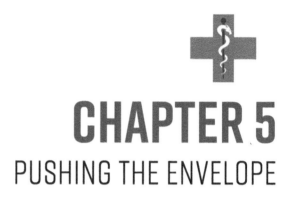

CHAPTER 5
PUSHING THE ENVELOPE

While we were making progress in turning RediClinic into a sustainable business, we had two fundamental problems that would be difficult to overcome. The first was that while RediClinics were generally profitable at the unit level, these profits were not sufficient to cover the corporate overhead necessary to support them. One of the drivers behind our initial push to grow rapidly was that it would enable us to leverage the corporate infrastructure over a large number of clinics. The problem with that strategy early on in the company's development was that we were not consistently generating profits at the unit level. Now we had the reverse problem—the clinics were profitable, but there weren't enough of them to support the overhead.

The second problem was that—without Revolution—we were depending on Walt and other angel investors to fund the company.

While these individual investors had been incredibly supportive, it didn't make sense for them to personally invest the kind of money it would take to grow RediClinic from its H-E-B base. That was why companies like RediClinic needed private equity and large strategic investors, and we didn't have any. I tried at various times to raise expansion capital from private equity funds, but they were generally in a "risk off" mode after the global financial crisis, and the offers to invest we received would have crushed the equity of our existing angel investors, which Walt and I were unwilling to do.

Joint ventures with health systems had enabled us to raise some expansion capital, but I felt that we needed to enhance our business in a way that would attract the kinds of investors we needed to grow and at a valuation that would be acceptable to our existing shareholders.

I had believed from the beginning that it made sense from a business and public health perspective for RediClinic to provide preventive care to our patients in addition to treating their acute/episodic conditions. As a result, RediClinic had always provided a more robust offering of screenings, medical tests, immunizations, and physicals than our competitors, which differentiated us to some extent and helped to reduce the cough-cold-flu seasonality of our core business.

We were constantly identifying and evaluating new services to offer, and there were two main criteria for green-lighting a new service. There had to be a proven demand for the new service among our primarily female customer base of "Soccer Moms," and a new service had to be capable of being consistently and professionally delivered by our APPs in a fifteen-minute visit. A surprising number of potential healthcare services didn't make the cut for one reason or another, but there was one service that continued to intrigue Danielle and me—weight management.

Clearly there was a consumer demand for weight management services, which companies like Weight Watchers and Jennie Craig had turned into a $40 billion U.S. market. We had also found that, consistent with national statistics, about 70 percent of RediClinic's patients were either overweight or obese, as measured by their body mass index, or BMI. Also, when we asked our patients what services they would like us to offer, weight management consistently ranked #1 on the list.

Just as importantly, extensive national research had irrefutably shown that obesity was a significant public health issue that was tied to increased morbidity and mortality, lower quality of life, and increased healthcare costs. Research at the time showed that obesity-related health issues accounted for more than 20 percent of all healthcare costs, a staggering $170 billion annually, and that healthcare costs for obese individuals were on average 40 percent higher than for normal-weight individuals. I thought that both our providers and third-party payors would support a RediClinic-branded weight management program if we could design one that was medically sound and effective and could be delivered at our clinics with online support.

While the weight management space was crowded, I believed we could grab a piece of the pie because there was a generally high level of consumer dissatisfaction with the results achieved through many of the commercially available programs where early weight loss was frequently followed by a disappointing rebound. Also, there were concerns about the long-term health impacts of the many programs that revolved around potentially dangerous appetite suppressants or meals-in-a-box that had limited, if any, nutritional value.

Furthermore, RediClinic had something going for it that no other weight management company could match: licensed healthcare professionals located in grocery stores who could draw large numbers of weight management patients from their existing patient panels and host stores' customers. Our grocery store locations also would enable program participants to conveniently purchase the food items they would need to follow our "real food" meal plans. Just as RediClinic's medical patients benefited from the convenience of our co-location with an in-store pharmacy, our weight loss patients could benefit from the convenience of having hundreds of nutritious, low-calorie grocery items just a few aisles away.

While our healthcare clinics located in grocery stores provided a natural advantage, I knew it was going to take a lot more than that for us to be successful in a highly competitive business in which we had little experience or credibility. We had to find a reputable medical director who would help us develop a medically supervised, real-food-based weight management program and who would be an effective spokesperson. After evaluating a number of potential candidates, we found exactly the right person in David Katz, MD-MPH.

David was an associate professor at the Yale University School of Medicine and the founder and director of the Yale-Griffin Prevention Research Center, which had been funded largely by the Centers for Disease Control and Prevention (CDC). He was—and is—an internationally recognized authority on diet, nutrition, and preventive medicine, having authored hundreds of peer-reviewed articles and nineteen books on these subjects. He was the subject matter expert we needed to develop our program, and he was excited about leveraging our clinics in grocery stores to create a unique program that would help patients to, as he put it, "lose weight while they were gaining health."

David brought a wealth of knowledge and experience to the task, including research he and his colleagues at Yale-Griffin had conducted that showed why people had so much trouble losing weight and keeping it off. They had found an astonishing 158 reasons behind long-term weight loss failure, compared to only seven reasons why individuals failed to quit smoking for good. These reasons ranged from lack of access to healthy foods—in neighborhoods known as "food deserts"—to sabotage from unsupportive family members. In addition, he had worked on a very ambitious project to score more than 100,000 grocery items based on their nutritional value. He understood exactly where our future weight management patients should go—and not go—in our host grocery stores to get the items they would need to achieve their weight loss and health improvement goals.

Danielle and I worked closely with David to develop what would be called the "Weigh Forward" program. It consisted of ten 15–20-minute visits at a RediClinic that were managed by one of our APPs. The first visit began with a basic physical exam and biometric testing to capture key measures such as blood pressure, cholesterol, hemoglobin A1c, and more. These baseline biometrics would enable us to track our patients' health gains, as well as their weight loss, as they progressed through the program. In addition to this medical aspect, Weigh Forward was designed to address three other key building blocks of sustained weight loss: behavior modification, diet/nutrition, and physical activity.

In order to compensate for the relatively brief duration of the in-clinic visits, we developed a comprehensive online complement available at myweighforward.com. This website provided Weigh Forward patients with access to a vast array of resources, including meal plans, recipes and shopping lists, progress trackers, e-coaching by diet/nutrition and fitness experts, community forums, blogs, reward programs, social networking connections to Facebook and Twitter, personalized push messaging, weekly nutrition tips, shopping and cooking guides with pictures, quick-tip slide shows on weight loss and related topics, videos featuring Dr. Katz for each visit, and fitness videos and plans for beginner, intermediate, and advanced patients. In addition to serving as a resource for our patients, there was a separate section on the website for APPs and ancillary clinic staff members that was designed and used for training purposes.

We knew from the beginning that the biggest challenge of Weigh Forward compared to many other programs was getting patients to stick with a real food program that didn't rely on drugs or packaged meals, but we also believed it would produce better long-term results if they did. To address this concern, we offered hundreds of meal plans that were low-calorie, nutritious, and family friendly; and to make them easier to prepare, we tried to limit the recipes to five ingredients or less and with a "door-to-table" preparation time of no more than thirty minutes. Nevertheless, we knew this wouldn't work for all patients all the time and that they would want access to meal and snack replacement products that would enable them to stick to the plan when they didn't have time to shop or cook.

Offering such products in our online store would not only improve patient adherence to the program, and thus weight loss success, but could also be an important source of revenue. The problem was that we couldn't find many off-the-shelf meal and snack replacement products that met our standards for caloric count and nutritional value and were also good-tasting and affordable enough that our patients would want to purchase and consume them. Many of the products we evaluated (mainly bars, shakes, soups, and "bites," which usually turned out to be processed foods packaged in small sizes) just didn't make the cut with David. By that time, Weigh Forward had become the first and only commercial weight management program to be accredited by the American College of Preventive Medicine

(ACPM), a prestigious medical society, so we had to meet their high standards as well.

We looked far and wide for products that met RediClinic's, David's, and ACPM's standards, but we didn't find many. Most of the products we evaluated either tasted like candy bars but were high in sugar, trans fats, or other unhealthy ingredients or contained healthy ingredients but tasted like sandpaper (or, as Danielle referred to it, "astronaut food"). Finding healthy and appetizing meal and snack replacement products was an ongoing challenge, but we figured we would eventually solve it and decided to launch with this part of the program still mostly a work in progress.

In retrospect, I would characterize the results from our first few months of Weigh Forward as mixed but promising. On the one hand, there was significant patient interest in the program and some great success stories. We had a couple of early patients who lost more than 70 pounds each and significantly improved their biometric markers in the process. They literally credited Weigh Forward with changing their lives where other programs had failed them completely. Many other patients lost 20 pounds or more in the first ten weeks (a healthy rate of weight loss) and signed up for our maintenance program.

On the other hand, while many of our APPs embraced Weigh Forward as an opportunity to help patients in more than a passing manner, others had trouble mixing our core acute/episodic visits—where diagnostic and treatment protocols were relatively straightforward—with the subtleties of weight management visits, which required coaching and knowledge transfer. In addition, it was clear that the online component of the program was very important to success and that it would have to be constantly expanded and refined to give our patients and APPs the support they needed.

There was also some consumer price resistance. We had initially priced the ten-week program at $499, or about $50 per visit, which was less than what we received for a typical office visit that usually took about the same amount of time. While some patients found this price to be very reasonable, others considered it too expensive. Therefore, we either had to find ancillary revenue streams (such as meal and snack replacement products) that would enable us to reduce the price of the program or had to get third-party payors to shoulder some of the cost. The rationale for the latter was sound given the mountains of research that conclusively showed that obesity led to both higher healthcare costs and reduced employee productivity. But getting payors to support a new kind of healthcare service required time and proven results, as we had learned in spades in the early days of RediClinic.

In one sense, however, the program almost immediately achieved one of our objectives, which was to heighten investor interest in our company. Other food and drug retailers we had been speaking with over the years about hosting RediClinics in their stores suddenly wanted to dig deeper. Also, private equity investors could see the potential of Weigh Forward not only as a differentiator for RediClinic but also as a program that could be licensed to other providers. These licensing prospects included primary care physicians who had the same high percentage of overweight and obese patients that we had but no way of helping them other than by referring them to weight loss programs that generally were neither effective nor medically sound.

Developing Weigh Forward had been a risky bet, but we had done it the right way and for the right reasons, and it looked like it just might pay off.

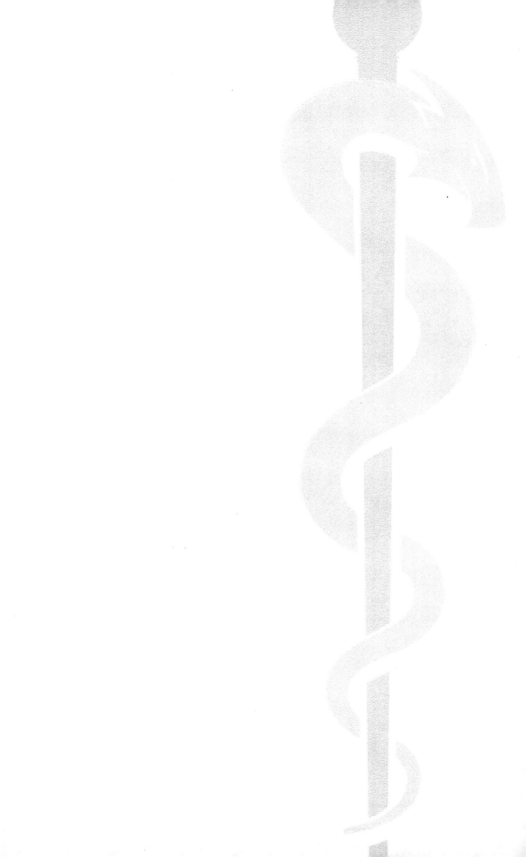

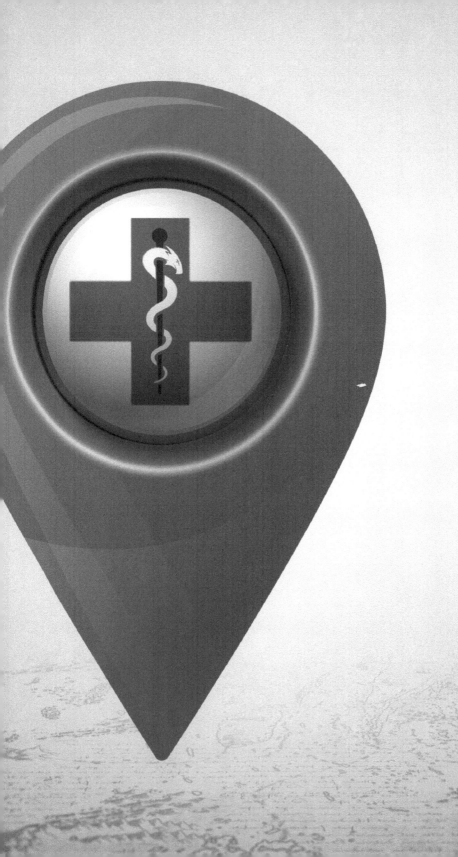

CHAPTER 6
SECURING A STRATEGIC INVESTOR

The three largest U.S. drugstore chains in 2013 were (and still are) CVS, Walgreens, and Rite Aid. Rite Aid was running last in this three-horse race, and they had experienced periodic financial challenges over the years. However, they seemed to be on the comeback trail, had generated more than $26 billion of revenues in 2012, and operated more than 5,000 stores nationwide. I had always favored grocery and big box stores as outlets for our clinics due to their higher foot traffic, but I believed we could be successful in drugstores if we operated in the highest volume ones and were located at the front of the stores where all shoppers could see us. In addition, I felt that Rite Aid would be a high-potential retail partner and possible investor if they followed CVS' and Walgreens' lead in seeking to transform their stores into healthcare destinations rather than just convenience stores with pharmacies.

The clinic decision-maker at Rite Aid was Robert Thompson, a company veteran who was their EVP of Pharmacy. I had met Robert when RediClinic was just getting off the ground and we were on a healthcare industry conference panel together about the future of retail clinics. The other panelist was Minute Clinic's then CEO, Michael Howe, who had previously been the CEO of Arby's. In response to an audience question about preventive services, Michael said that he didn't see much potential in them. I challenged his position on this, expressing my view that preventive services should be offered not only because this would enable retail clinics to satisfy an important but largely unmet public health need but also because they had value in reducing the seasonality of retail clinics' core acute/episodic services. When Robert piped up to agree with me, I knew we were on the same page, and we had subsequently developed a friendship.

However, Rite Aid had developed an early partnership with Take Care, so I didn't see much opportunity with them, and we didn't have the bandwidth anyway as we were still focused on expanding with Duane Reade, Walmart, H-E-B, and Walgreens. Still, I made a point of staying in touch with Robert, and one day a few years after we had met he called to say that Take Care had abruptly pulled out of Rite Aid's stores in the Seattle-Tacoma area and to ask whether RediClinic would be interested in stepping into their shoes. We had our hands full at the time, but I respected Robert and appreciated his offering us this opportunity, so I agreed to take a closer look. A few weeks later, I traveled to Seattle-Tacoma to meet with Robert and tour a few of the stores and clinics that Take Care had evacuated.

The meeting with Robert was productive, and the Seattle-Tacoma area was booming, but I couldn't figure out why Take Care had exited. I knew that they were trying to expand their partnership with Walgreens, so it was possible that competitive conflict had been the main cause, but I wondered whether the poor performance of their clinics had been a contributing factor as well. During my tour, I sensed that customer volumes in the host Rite Aid stores were not particularly strong, and market research revealed that the prevalence of Health Maintenance Organizations (HMOs) in the Pacific Northwest—which provide insurance and care in a closed system—would make it hard for us to gain in-network status with many of the largest payors.

We also found that there was a shortage of APPs in the state of Washington, which suggested that our labor costs would be higher than in other markets. For these reasons, as well as the fact that we were already juggling a lot of balls in a still unproven business, I reluctantly told Robert that while I appreciated the opportunity, we had decided to pass. He was gracious about it but clearly frustrated by the combination of Take Care's exit and our disinterest. I thought the Rite Aid door might be closed forever.

The subsequent combination of factors that caused RediClinic to retreat to Texas and H-E-B had changed the picture for us entirely, so I continued to stay in touch with Robert. Also, our financial results had improved, and we had launched the Weigh Forward program with some early success. I still had reservations about the drugstore venue being the right place for RediClinic as an independent business, but it would make a lot more sense if Rite Aid owned the company and used it to enhance their stores' overall performance. This was the way that CVS was using Minute Clinic and Walgreens was using Take Care. Drugstores also were not as strong a venue for Weigh Forward as grocery stores, but they might work if Rite Aid was willing to stock the front end of their stores with more healthy items.

Meanwhile, the picture had changed for Rite Aid as well. Under CEO John Standley's leadership, Rite Aid's financial performance had improved significantly. In 2013, their stock price went up over 250 percent within a few months, making it one of the top performing stocks of the year. The company had more financial flexibility as a result, and I thought Rite Aid might expand in the retail clinic space since their two largest competitors were moving forward aggressively to open clinics in their stores. My hunch proved to be correct when Robert called me to request information about RediClinic's recent financial performance and future plans. When I asked him why they wanted this information, he said that it was in connection with their possible interest in partnering with RediClinic and possibly acquiring the company.

This was an exciting possibility, but in the interest of always wanting to have more than one bidder, we had been exploring transactions with a number of other potential investors, including one that couldn't have been more different from Rite Aid. In our endless search for low-calorie and nutritious meal and snack replacement products that tasted good and were affordable, we were introduced to a company then called MBX, which was backed by an experienced and very successful private investor, Peter Castleman. Peter had been the chairman and managing partner of J.H. Whitney & Co., the country's first venture capital firm and coincidentally a minority investor in Playback Associates when I had worked there in the mid-1970s. He had spent twenty years at J.H. Whitney before retiring to form a successful family office called Westwind Investors.

Westwind had partnered with a talented food scientist to create MBX, an innovative line of meal and food replacement products that met all of Weigh Forward's criteria. Their products were made from thirty-four natural nutrients that they claimed were essential to healthy weight loss. We were excited to find MBX and believed that offering their product line would help Weigh Forward patients adhere to our program while providing a significant additional source of revenue. Peter and his MBX colleagues, in turn, seemed to be excited about the Weigh Forward program, its association with Dr. David Katz, and the potential to combine our program with MBX products to create a global weight management brand.

By the time Robert had expressed Rite Aid's serious interest in RediClinic, we had entered into discussions with Peter about spinning off Weigh Forward in conjunction with a Westwind investment or even Westwind purchasing all of RediClinic. This was an appealing alternative to Rite Aid in many respects, although I was concerned that Peter—with his deep background as a successful investor in early-stage companies—might undervalue our core assets to the point that the transaction wouldn't make sense for many of our shareholders.

With this going on in the background, our discussions and information sharing with Rite Aid had reached the point where Robert invited Walt, Danielle, and me to present to John Standley and the rest of Rite Aid's executive management team at their corporate headquarters in Camp Hill, Pennsylvania, just across the Susquehanna River from the state capital in Harrisburg. I had visited Rite Aid's headquarters a number of times, almost always staying in Harrisburg because it had one of the better hotels in the area, and I enjoyed running along the river and across a short bridge to a small state park called City Island.

I can remember running with Danielle in City Park early in the morning before the presentation and realizing halfway through that the future of RediClinic might depend upon the meeting we were about to have and the presentation we were about to give. At that moment, I decided to ditch the slides we had prepared and instead rely on our unmatched depth of retail clinic experience to carry the day.

As it turned out, it did, or at least it got us a lot closer to a deal. John and his team were very attentive. I began with an overview of RediClinic, our experience, and our future plans. We then spent the rest of the time responding very effectively, I thought, to all of their questions. It was a performance that could only have been the by-product of a team that had been truly battle-tested and knew every detail of its business because its survival had depended upon it. John and his team didn't make any definitive commitments during the meeting, but I knew we had given it our best effort. I had come to believe over the years that this is all you can do in business and in life. Do your best. Control what you can control. And leave the rest to a higher authority.

As I had hoped and expected, Robert called the next day to say that they were serious about acquiring RediClinic and wanted to start negotiating the price and key terms to be included in a letter of intent (LOI). One of the challenges of the price negotiation was that all our clinics were located in a state where Rite Aid had no stores, so they were essentially buying the modest profits from these units along with a proven retail clinic business and operating model (RediClinic had managed more than three million patient visits by then without any safety issues), an unproven new service in Weigh Forward, and an experienced management team. Another challenge was that there was a clause in our master agreement with H-E-B that enabled them to terminate all our leases upon a change of control, which an acquisition by Rite Aid would trigger.

We were able to hold out for a good price, partially because we had more confidence in the business now that it was moving toward enterprise profitability, and because other parties were interested, but there were many tense moments in the negotiation because we knew in our hearts that Rite Aid was probably our best option.

Once the LOI had been negotiated and signed, Rite Aid's due diligence team swung into action. Very few members of the Redi-Clinic team had experienced the thoroughness of a Fortune 500 company's due diligence process, and most of them won't likely want to again. Rite Aid's team was not only very professional but also very large and extraordinarily thorough. We referred to them cordially as the "Mongol Hordes" and at one meeting gave all of them T-shirts displaying a well-known depiction of the real ones. I frequently wondered whether our small company would be able to withstand this level of scrutiny, but in the end, the investments we had made in creating the infrastructure for a company that had been designed to scale—and had been scaled in the past—enabled us to pass muster.

I remember one particularly touching and encouraging moment after Rite Aid's due diligence team had finished their work and left our offices for the last time to be taken back to the airport by our loyal and quite elderly car service driver, Julia Hatch. Julia was a reliable chauffeur who drove an aging Chevy suburban that was on its last legs. She never said much but couldn't help but have overheard a lot about RediClinic's twisted path from the many cell phone calls I made and received as she shuttled me back and forth from the Houston airport over a period of many years. After dropping the Rite Aid team off at the airport, she called me from her car—the only time she ever did this—to tell me that they said good things about RediClinic and our team, and it sounded to her like they were committed to some kind of transaction with us.

While this was promising, we still had a few more hurdles to clear. The biggest was convincing H-E-B that they should approve our pending change of control rather than exercise their option to terminate our leases. Our rationale was that they should do it because Rite Aid wasn't a competitive threat. Also, we argued, RediClinic would be more stable with a large investor behind it, and, perhaps most importantly, Rite Aid would be willing to invest in RediClinic's continued growth in Texas.

I wondered whether investing in Texas would prove to be the case given Rite Aid's stated priority to open RediClinics in hundreds of their stores elsewhere, but we eventually got H-E-B over the line just before Danielle, Stephen Payne, our very able CFO at the time, and I were set to meet with John and others at Rite Aid's annual vendor meeting in Las Vegas. I know many people like Vegas, but I'm not one of them. I'm not a gambler, at least in the casino sense of the term, and the man-made plasticity of the environment doesn't appeal to me. However, I was happy to make this trip.

After a full day of meetings with Robert and other Rite Aid executives, I was ushered into CEO John Standley's enormous suite at the Bellagio to meet with him and his EVP of human resources. The meeting was primarily focused on our path forward together, and I knew we finally had a deal when John arranged for me and my team to be chauffeured back to the airport in a car that was a lot fancier than what I was used to with Julia. A new chapter was about to begin with little RediClinic as a wholly owned subsidiary of a very large corporation.

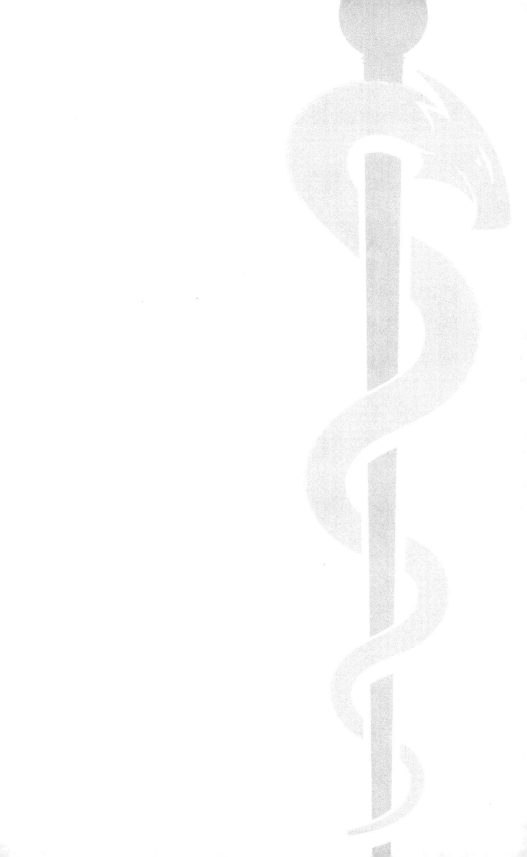

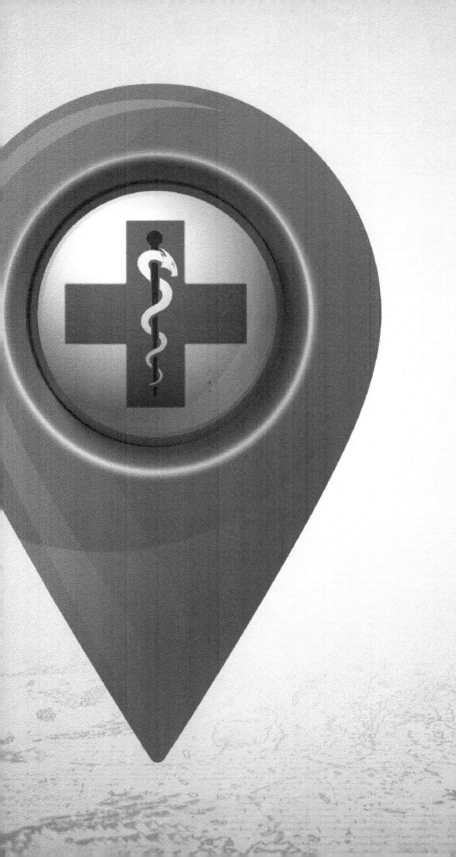

CHAPTER 7
FROM ENTREPRENEUR TO CORPORATE EXECUTIVE

I suspected that the transition to corporate life would be challenging for me after more than twenty-five years of entrepreneurship, but I was excited about the opportunity to scale RediClinic again, build Weigh Forward, and avoid having to do it all on a shoestring. It was also a great relief to have monetized the investments of the many angels (truly!) who had supported RediClinic over the years. They had stuck with us through the company's many twists and turns, and I had spent many sleepless nights wondering whether their investments would ever pay off or even be recouped.

But it didn't take very long for me to realize that I wasn't in Kansas anymore! Almost immediately, Rite Aid insisted upon redesigning RediClinic's logo and changing its color scheme (which was used not only in the logo but in all our clinics and marketing materials) from our original orange and teal to the green and blue color scheme that Rite Aid had recently adopted. While Rite Aid's marketing department did a great job on the redesign, and their real estate department subsequently did a great job constructing our new clinics, the result was that RediClinics were now going to look different in Rite Aid stores outside of Texas than they had looked in H-E-B and other retailers' stores for close to a decade. As there was no money to retrofit our Texas clinics with the new logo and color scheme, we now effectively had two brands. This would make it more difficult for us to build a national brand in Rite Aid, H-E-B, and other retailers' stores, which I had been given the assurance we would be able to do.

The next big decision, also made without much input from our team, was that we would begin opening RediClinics in Rite Aid stores in Philadelphia, New Jersey, and (you guessed it) Seattle-Tacoma, where I had declined to open them when we were independent due to concerns about their financial viability in this market. I was supportive of Philadelphia because Rite Aid was the #1 drugstore chain there, and we had many stores to choose from. In the other two markets, where Rite Aid did not have as strong a presence, I agreed on the condition that we attempt to secure a large health system partner in each market. This would enable us to share the financial risk while ensuring our success by leveraging our partners' local brand awareness, piggybacking on their typically higher reimbursement rates, and benefiting from utilization by their employees and patient referrals from their affiliated physicians.

John, Robert, and other senior Rite Aid executives did not completely understand the health system partnering model RediClinic had developed over the previous few years, though they were aware that we had entered into a joint venture with Seton Healthcare in

Austin, Texas, a short time before our acquisition by Rite Aid. I was able to convince them that this was a good model for us to employ in markets where we had concerns about RediClinic's ability to achieve stand-alone profitability in a short period of time. We all understood that the clinics' contribution to their host stores' overall financial performance was paramount, but I didn't want to start my career at Rite Aid by opening too many new clinics at one time that could result in a significant cash drain. Fortunately, we were able to find two excellent joint venture partners in Hackensack-Meridian Health in New Jersey and MultiCare in Seattle-Tacoma.

The next shoe to drop was Rite Aid's insistence that RediClinics be located in the back of their stores, closer to the pharmacies, rather than in the front where all shoppers would see them when they entered. Rite Aid's rationale for this was that the proximity to the pharmacy would increase the likelihood that patients would choose to have their prescriptions filled at the in-store pharmacy. They also believed that the location of their pharmacies in the back of their stores had not negatively impacted sales and so reasoned that it would be the same for our clinics.

My counterargument was that the vast majority of patients would choose to have their prescriptions filled at the in-store pharmacy even if RediClinics were located in the front of the store, because it would still be far more convenient than having to make a separate trip to another pharmacy. More than 85 percent of our patients in H-E-B and Walmart stores voluntarily filled their prescriptions at the in-store pharmacies even though we were located at the front of these stores, and the distance to the pharmacies in the back was far longer in a grocery or big box store than it would be in Rite Aid's much smaller stores.

Furthermore, I argued that drugstore shoppers had been conditioned over time to know that there was a pharmacy in the back of the store, whereas they might not expect to find a healthcare clinic located there. Given the relatively low foot traffic in many Rite Aid stores, I argued further, we needed to be near the front of the store where everyone could see us. I might have added that removing a few aisles of Cokes, M&Ms, and potato chips from the front of the store—or moving these unhealthy items to the back—to make room for a RediClinic might be a good trade-off from both a public health and a financial perspective, but I didn't want to gore too many oxen so early on in my new corporate career. In any case, my arguments fell on deaf ears, and RediClinics were thereafter relegated to the back of Rite Aid stores.

Despite these early challenges, my team was excited to be on the growth path again, not only in Rite Aid stores but also with other retailers in markets where Rite Aid did not operate. While focusing mainly on growth within Rite Aid, I didn't want to give up on the grocery store venue where we had achieved success with H-E-B and where I felt Weigh Forward would have a better chance of stand-alone financial success. In this regard, we had been chasing the large grocery chain, Safeway, for some time, partially because we had noticed that they were building elaborate spaces near the pharmacies in many of their stores that seemed like they had been designed to be occupied by clinics.

However, we didn't seem to be making much progress with Safeway despite many seemingly promising meetings with senior executives. As it turned out, Safeway had other plans for those new clinic spaces. Safeway's then CEO, Steve Burd, with whom I had spoken about RediClinic, had made the unfathomable decision to spend a reported $350 million to build out eight hundred spaces in Safeway stores where he intended to offer the ill-fated Theranos blood testing system, even though Safeway had not reached a definitive agreement with the company. In any case, Theranos' technology never lived up to the fraudulent claims of its founders, causing huge financial losses for Theranos investors and a prison sentence for its founder, Elizabeth Holmes.

The biggest disappointment of my early days at Rite Aid was that management did not treat Weigh Forward as a priority. This was difficult to understand, as Rite Aid executives had assigned a meaningful amount of value to it in the price paid to acquire RediClinic. While I understood the importance of focusing on RediClinic's core business, I felt that it was a mistake to neglect Weigh Forward due to its potentially positive impact on both RediClinic and Rite Aid.

We tried to keep Weigh Forward alive by working with Rite Aid's front-end merchants to stock the shelves with healthier items that would be compatible with our meal plans. We also introduced Rite Aid to Peter Castleman in hopes that he could interest them in carrying a line of MBX products. Unfortunately, none of this worked, mainly because Rite Aid's convenience store culture had not fully embraced the idea of their stores as healthcare destinations—which CVS had evidenced their intention to do by ceasing to sell cigarettes in their stores.

Another missed opportunity was in telemedicine, now commonly referred to as "virtual care." Long before COVID-19 put virtual care on the healthcare map for good, I had believed that it would become a permanent part of the healthcare delivery landscape, primarily due to its convenience for patients and the increasing capabilities and decreasing costs of the technologies required to implement it. Telemedicine's convenience and easy application to the kind of basic healthcare RediClinic offered made it a perfect fit as an additional channel through which we could provide accessible and affordable care. As a result, we had kept a close watch on its continued development.

Shortly before Rite Aid had acquired us, Robert had entered into an agreement with a young company called HealthSpot to test their telemedicine kiosk in a few Rite Aid stores in Ohio. HealthSpot's kiosk was a small, self-contained shell (we referred to it as a "space capsule") that could accommodate one patient at a time and was outfitted with a number of medical devices that enabled the patient to facilitate a correct diagnosis by the on-screen provider. These included a blood pressure cuff and stethoscope that the patient could self-administer at the provider's direction and a high-definition camera that could be pointed by the patient at physical areas of diagnostic relevance, such as an ear, throat, or skin rash. The results of the pilot had been generally positive, with the main complaint having to do with the delay between the time the patient inside the kiosk requested a provider visit and when the provider appeared on screen to attend to them.

I thought the kiosk had great potential as a RediClinic-branded service for several reasons. First, it was consistent with our mission to provide accessible and affordable care. Second, the kiosks were small enough to fit in stores that didn't have space for a clinic or whose traffic couldn't justify one. They could also be placed at schools, worksites, and other non-retail venues. And third, the kiosks could be supported by RediClinic's hundreds of APPs, who could serve as virtual providers when not treating patients in one of our clinics, thereby increasing labor productivity and company profitability. In addition, the kiosks would be a low-cost solution because they only required a single nonprofessional attendant to be on site, to collect payment at the time of service and introduce patients to the easy-to-use functionality of the kiosk.

This all made sense except for the fact that HealthSpot's founder had unrealistic expectations about the value of his company if we wanted to acquire it and on the financial terms if we wanted to license the kiosks on a semi-exclusive basis. Nevertheless, I thought there was a deal to be made. However, it wasn't clear that I was authorized to take the lead in negotiating one, nor was it clear which Rite Aid business unit or department would own the kiosks if we were successful.

There were too many other Rite Aid executives in the mix with no clear lines of authority. As a result, no deal was ever consummated while I was with the company, and the opportunity was missed for both RediClinic and Rite Aid. As a postscript, I was told that Rite Aid eventually purchased HealthSpot out of bankruptcy a few years later, but by that time the opportunity had been squandered and HealthSpot's technology had become obsolete due to inattention and lack of funds. So, the kiosks were "virtually" worthless.

Despite these disappointments and false steps on the business front, Rite Aid was providing plenty of support to me personally. A few months after the acquisition, Robert asked if I would also run another company they had acquired called Health Dialog, an early innovator in what was then referred to as "care management" and is now known as "population health management." Health Dialog's main business was contracting with health plans to identify and provide support to their chronically ill members and those predicted to fall into this category soon. The company assisted in areas like medication adherence, diet/nutrition, and physical activity, with the goal of helping to improve the quality of their members' lives while reducing the disproportionally high healthcare costs that were incurred by this cohort.

Health Dialog's service had been built around a proprietary "Care Pathways" model that enabled them to identify a payor's current and future high-cost members from an analysis of huge amounts of claims and other data. They also maintained a robust patient outreach program, which was mostly telephonic and staffed primarily with highly trained registered nurses. While the company's telephonic platform had worked well during its formative stages in the early 2000s, consumers' increasing reluctance to answer calls from unknown persons had progressively limited Health Dialog's ability to interact frequently enough with targeted members to the point where the cost-effectiveness of Health Dialog's service was being challenged by its largest customers.

It was clear to me that the solution to this was to create a digital platform that would complement Health Dialog's telephonic/print platform. A digital platform would make it easier for members to interact on their own time, and it would enable Health Dialog to expand the tools at its disposal to achieve their clients' health improvement and cost reduction objectives. It was telling, of course, that the nation's largest third-party payors had to hire companies like Health Dialog to provide disease and lifestyle management support, which arguably should have been provided by hospitals, physician practices, and other traditional providers who were interacting with these patients on a regular basis.

Understanding what needed to be done at Health Dialog and executing on this vision, however, were two very different things. Creating the kind of digital platform that would be necessary for Health Dialog to compete against sophisticated new population health management players was a significant undertaking, especially given the company's shrinking revenues and Rite Aid's general lack of technology expertise. Rite Aid had antiquated legacy systems in many areas of its business and had employed at least three chief information officers (CIOs) during my tenure at the company. These included one CIO who left after only three weeks on the job, reportedly telling some of his colleagues—as he was heading out the door—that he hadn't realized how big a job it would be to bring Rite Aid's systems into the twenty-first century.

Nevertheless, I liked Health Dialog's business and its team members and believed that the company served a valuable purpose. I moved forward as aggressively as I could to begin building the new "Interact" platform, with technology support from an outside vendor. I also worked diligently to minimize Health Dialog's revenue decline in its traditional disease management, twenty-four-hour nurse line, and "shared decision-making" businesses. The latter business line revolved around the sale to payors of proprietary patient education videos from a large but dated library that had proven effective at educating members about their treatment options, frequently resulting in the delay of costly and unnecessary surgeries. This new encounter with condition- and procedure-related point-of-care videos harkened back to my days at American Medical Communications!

While the effort I put into Health Dialog was gratifying, and our team was reasonably successful in reviving the company's fortunes in a relatively short period of time, it came at a cost to RediClinic. I was not able to focus as much attention on it as I probably should have, and both Danielle and our good new CFO, Jeff Fields, had been drawn into the management of Health Dialog, as well, because I needed their support to do both of my jobs. While it was a compliment that Rite Aid's management had asked me to run two companies, it may not have been in the best interests of either one that I had to split my time, focus, and energy between them. This was particularly true because both companies had significant but different challenges to address and opportunities to capitalize on.

Then, one day, everything changed. I had traveled to Rite Aid's headquarters in Camp Hill to make a presentation to Rite Aid's board on our progress with RediClinic. Arriving on the executive floor where the board room was located, I was told by John's assistant that the meeting agenda had changed due to an "unanticipated development." She situated me in a small conference room where I broke out my laptop and started grinding through my emails. I checked with her periodically to find out when she thought I would be called into the meeting, but she had no idea. After a couple hours, John appeared in my conference room with a big smile on his face. He told me that Rite Aid had entered into a definitive agreement to merge with (read "be acquired by") Walgreens. He then ushered me into the board meeting, where I finally gave my presentation. It went smoothly, though it was apparent that the directors' thoughts were understandably elsewhere.

As I learned more details about the transaction, it was clear that it would be good for my bank account, at least in the short term. Walgreens was proposing to pay a significant premium over the strike prices of the Rite Aid stock options and restricted shares I had been granted. However, I knew that the "merger" would not be good news for RediClinic because Walgreens had acquired Take Care and was already moving forward to open clinics in many of their stores. I also had no idea whether Walgreens would be interested in Health Dialog, particularly since it was in turnaround mode. In any case, I had no choice but to do what I could to reassure the teams at both companies and dive into the integration process that began almost immediately after the merger announcement under the auspices of Walgreens' version of the "Mongol Hordes."

Over the following months, several things happened that made me start to wonder whether Rite Aid was the right place for me. The first was that Rite Aid's senior management started pulling back on many growth initiatives, including some that were related to Redi-Clinic and Health Dialog. This is a common reaction among companies that are being acquired, and the logic is threefold. First, it doesn't make sense to make investments in the future when the company is not likely to be around long enough to benefit from them. Second, forward-looking initiatives might not be consistent with the acquiring company's strategy. And third, eliminating expenses related to these initiatives improves near-term financial results, which can help to seal the deal at the agreed-upon acquisition price or an even higher one. While all of these made sense, my experience had taught me that if you're not growing, you're dying, and the entrepreneur still in me didn't want to sit idle for too long.

> MY EXPERIENCE HAD TAUGHT ME THAT IF YOU'RE NOT GROWING, YOU'RE DYING, AND THE ENTREPRENEUR STILL IN ME DIDN'T WANT TO SIT IDLE FOR TOO LONG.

The second thing that happened was that it became clear that federal government approval of the Walgreens-Rite Aid transaction was far from assured and that in any case the process was likely to play out over an extended period of time. The back story here is that corporate transactions over a certain dollar threshold must secure antitrust clearance under the Hart-Scott-Rodino Act from either the Federal Trade Commission (FTC) or the Justice Department.

Because the Walgreens-Rite Aid initial transaction value of $17 billion was well over the threshold, both parties had to provide detailed information to the lead investigator, which in this case was the FTC. This usually occurred when the definitive agreement was reached between the parties but before the deal had formally closed. The FTC then had thirty days to review the information and either stay silent, which was tantamount to approval, or request the "additional information" they deemed necessary to further their evaluation.

As expected by the parties given the magnitude of the transaction and the fact that it would create the largest drugstore chain in the United States with more than 12,000 stores nationwide and dominant positions in many markets, the FTC issued first one and then multiple requests for additional information. Each of these successive requests was extensive and required armies of lawyers and consultants at both companies to devote significant amounts of time to prepare their responses. Upon receipt of the responses to their most recent information request, the FTC again had thirty days to respond, or not, but at every turn, they could and did move the proverbial goal posts by asking for more information. The result of this iterative process was that the parties concluded—a full two years after the HSR process had begun—that FTC approval of the merger would not be forthcoming. They jointly announced that they were going to drop their merger plans and instead seek approval for another transaction that called for Rite Aid to sell half of its stores to Walgreens for a significantly reduced amount.

Recognizing that this was not going to sit well with many of its executives who had essentially been treading water for the previous two years, Rite Aid's management implemented a retention plan designed to keep me and others around while the company did a reset. By that time, however, I wasn't sure if I was up for it.

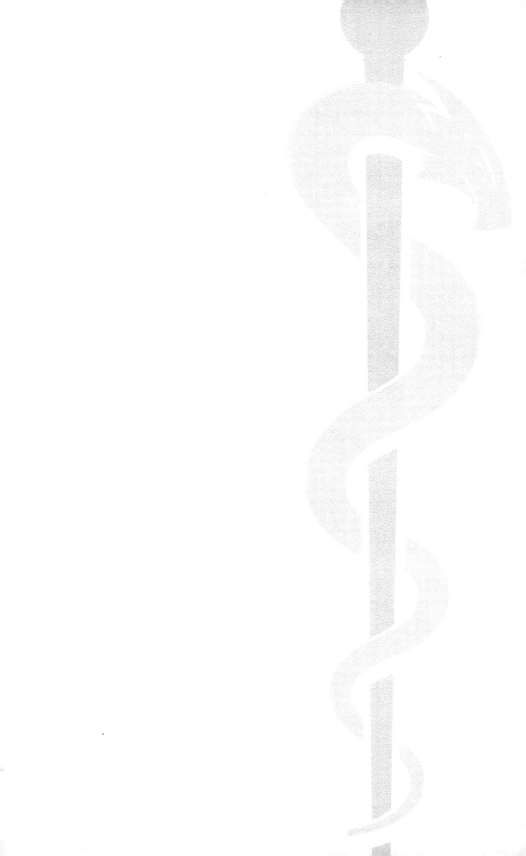

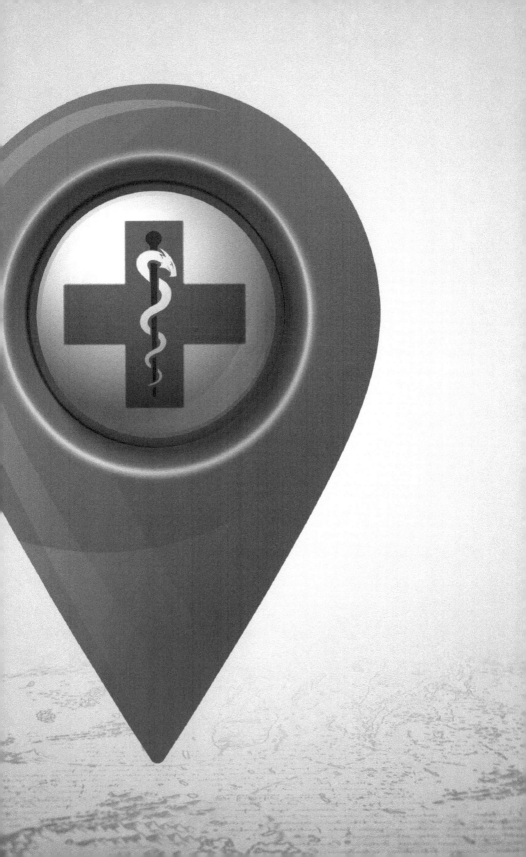

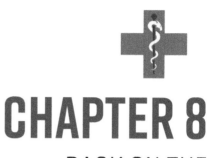

CHAPTER 8

BACK ON THE
ENTREPRENEURIAL TRAIL

Facing the prospect of resurrecting RediClinic and Health Dialog from their merger-induced slumbers in the context of a smaller Rite Aid that was under renewed financial pressure, I reluctantly began thinking about whether this was the right spot for me. I had always been up for a challenge, but it wasn't at all clear that transforming Rite Aid into a healthcare company was still a strategic imperative or whether the company had the necessary resources even if it was. Under these circumstances, I sensed that turning RediClinic into a national brand and reinventing Health Dialog as a market-leading population health management company would be almost impossible.

While these thoughts were percolating in the back of my mind, I got a call one day from Spencer Stuart, a leading executive search firm I had engaged to recruit executives for my previous companies. They asked if I would be interested in considering the possibility of becoming the CEO of an urgent care provider called FastMed. Very coincidentally (or was it fate?), John Standley had asked me to explore the possibility of acquiring FastMed and merging it into RediClinic shortly after I started at Rite Aid. While we ultimately did not make an offer to acquire the company, I had been impressed with FastMed from reviewing their materials, meeting with management at their corporate offices in Raleigh, North Carolina, and visiting a few of their clinics.

FastMed had been an early entrant in the urgent care business at about the same time I co-founded RediClinic. While urgent care clinics and RediClinics generally filled the same need—to provide consumers with easy access to basic healthcare—there were important differences between the two delivery models. Because retail-based clinics were located inside other stores, they were smaller than stand-alone urgent care clinics and had a more limited scope of practice. This was mainly because host retailers had limited space for leasing to third-party tenants and didn't want patients with more serious medical conditions dripping blood or demonstrating other signs of medical distress in their stores.

The smaller size of retail-based clinics limited the number of patients they could handle compared to larger, stand-alone urgent care clinics. In addition, urgent care clinics could generate higher average revenue per patient visit than retail-based clinics because urgent care clinics could treat patients who needed higher levels of care. On the other hand, the co-location of retail-based clinics with in-store pharmacies maximized convenience for patients, and retail-based clinics' exposure to hundreds and even thousands of daily shoppers and employees in their host stores minimized the need for the levels of advertising and other forms of promotion that urgent cares generally required. In other words, FastMed and RediClinic were essentially serving the same consumer need for access to affordable, basic healthcare, though their delivery models had relative advantages and disadvantages.

The prospect of leaving RediClinic and, in particular, Danielle and many others who had been with me throughout the many twists and turns of the company was difficult to contemplate. However, I knew myself well enough to realize that I wouldn't be happy or productive in a no-growth mode and that the entrepreneur in me was increasingly frustrated by the politics and bureaucracy of corporate life. Understanding that many of my teammates probably felt the same way, I also thought that eventually I might be able to take some of them with me, wherever I landed. So, I figured—what the heck—why not explore the opportunity at FastMed?

After a series of meetings with Spencer Stuart, they set up a meeting for me with Kip Turco, the operating partner responsible for FastMed at Abry Partners, a well-respected private equity firm that had purchased the company two years earlier. Kip and I hit it off immediately. He was a no bullshit guy with deep operating experience and had been parachuted into FastMed when the company had begun to falter. As he described the situation to me, it was clear that FastMed was a reclamation project. At this point, all but one member of the company's senior management team had "resigned;" its operating and financial results were in the tank, and Kip was effectively running the company. He believed I was the right person to turn FastMed around, but he needed to fill the empty CEO slot quickly, and it didn't take long for Abry to make me an offer.

The offer was, on balance, very fair. There were a few details to be worked out, but Kip and I were able to resolve them quickly, so now I had to decide. I was on my way to attend a two-day, off-site Rite

Aid strategic planning meeting when Kip made his final offer. I told him that I needed to participate in the Rite Aid meeting but that I would get back to him soon afterward with my decision. In addition to feeling that it was too late to pull out of the meeting, which was designed to set Rite Aid's go-forward strategy, I also thought it would be a good opportunity to see what the future might bring if I stayed put at Rite Aid.

By that time, I was reporting directly to CEO John Standley and was one of approximately twenty executives invited to the meeting. The meeting was productive, and parts of it were even fun, as I had gotten to know many of the other Rite Aid executives, and both respected them and enjoyed their company. However, I didn't believe that the company was committed to the kind of transformation I thought would be required to reinvigorate it, and I wasn't confident that I would be able to do more than influence it on the margins. Not that I doubted John's leadership, as he was a very talented executive, but we didn't share the same vision.

On the way back to the airport after the meeting, I reflected on a phrase I had come back to many times over the years: "Here Be Dragons." I had first learned of this phrase and the story behind it from a *Newsweek* editorial by J. Lipton:

Centuries ago, when a cartographer ran out of known world before he ran out of parchment, he inscribed the words "here be dragons" at the edge of the ominously blank terra incognita, a signal to the voyager that he entered the unknown region at his peril. But for some, like Columbus and Magellan, the warning seems not to have been a deterrent but a goad.

In his editorial, Lipton continued:

> Long before Columbus probed the world's edge, the Chinese, seeking an ideograph to represent the turning point we call "crisis" in English, performed a miracle of linguistic compression by combining two existing characters, the symbol for "opportunity" and the symbol for "danger" to create the character "wei-ji," which stands as an eternal assertion that, since opportunity and danger are inseparable, it is impossible to make a significant forward move without encountering danger: and, obversely, the scent of danger should alert us to the fact that we may be headed in the right direction.[8]

Sensing both danger and opportunity, I decided to jump into the FastMed fire.

I called Kip to accept the offer and then faced the very emotional task of informing Danielle, Jeff Fields, and others who worked closely with me at RediClinic and Health Dialog, as well as John Standley and others at Rite Aid (Robert Thompson had retired by then), that I was moving on. Everyone was supportive, but I could tell they felt to varying degrees that I was abandoning them, and the long farewell tour was draining. Despite this, and even though I was leaving some retention bonus money on the table at Rite Aid by departing before the year-end payout, I felt a surge of energy and excitement about the new FastMed challenge ahead.

My first days at FastMed in November 2017 were unsettling, to say the least. I met Kip and one of his colleagues from Abry Partners at

---

8   James Lipton, "My Turn," *Newsweek*, December 6, 1976.

my hotel in Scottsdale, Arizona, and traveled with them to FastMed's offices in the nearby Phoenix suburb of Gilbert. The previous CEO had recently moved the company's corporate offices and much of its senior management team from North Carolina to Arizona, which seemed like an odd decision because North Carolina was where the company had been founded, where it operated more than fifty clinics, and where it enjoyed strategic support from its first major investor, Blue Cross Blue Shield of North Carolina. Arizona, conversely, was where it operated just twenty-five clinics, most of which were struggling financially due to unfavorable reimbursement rates from legacy payor contracts. The relocation decision by itself had seemed somewhat suspect, but when I arrived at the company's offices to find they were in a building that otherwise doubled as a rentable wedding venue, I started to wonder what I had gotten myself into.

There was no time for second-guessing, however, as the company was in trouble and needed a new strategy and plan to start digging out. The most obvious symptom of FastMed's difficulties was that its more than ninety clinics in North Carolina, Arizona, and Texas had experienced month-over-month patient visit volume declines for each of the past fifteen months. In a business like RediClinic that was highly dependent upon consistently high patient volumes to cover fixed labor costs, this was causing financial issues and suggested that patients generally didn't like the service they were receiving.

Upon closer inspection, I thought I could see the root cause of the problem. As a cost-cutting measure, the former management team had implemented an inflexible labor model that required all clinics to be staffed with no more than three individuals (whom I started referring to as "team members" rather than employees)—one APP, one medical assistant, and one front-desk assistant. The predictable result of this rigid policy was that there were long lines at the most successful clinics, which historically had generated most of the company's profits.

Because "wait time" is the single biggest patient dissatisfier in retail medicine, this led to patient abandonment and poor social media reviews. Inadequate staffing also led to disgruntled staff in the clinics because they were overwhelmed with angry patients and didn't feel as if they had the ability to be successful. Some of the providers with the largest and most loyal patient followings had left the company, and I could tell from early clinic visits that others were considering it.

The obvious remedial strategy was to introduce a more flexible labor model that was based on supporting both current and historical clinic volumes, which I implemented immediately. It was a good start and produced almost immediately positive results, but I knew that much more would be required to turn the ship around and begin to realize what I viewed as FastMed's tremendous but as yet unrealized potential.

The next order of business was to transform the company's culture, which in my mind required two key changes. The first was that everyone in the company who was not directly involved in patient care—including me—needed to realize that our patient-facing team members were the key to FastMed's success. Our main job, in what I now referred to as "Support Services," was to support them, directly or indirectly.

More than 80 percent of the company's workforce was located in clinics spread over three nonadjacent states, and I knew from my RediClinic experience that team members who worked long hours in these thinly staffed clinics had an understandable tendency to become lonely and frustrated if they didn't feel properly appreciated and supported. Prompt and effective responses to clinic team members' ongoing requests for help in areas like facilities maintenance, information technology, and medical records were essential to improving their work experience and giving them the support they needed to provide superior service and care to our patients.

The second aspect of the cultural transformation was to make FastMed more mission driven. Having led RediClinic, Health Dialog, and previous health-related companies, as well as from my own personal experience, I knew that people are attracted to work in healthcare because they want to help people live happier and healthier lives. If they think management believes that it's all about the money, they will become disengaged and it will be difficult to attract, motivate, and retain the kinds of individuals it takes to make companies like FastMed successful. In FastMed's case, the company had a mission, but no one seemed to know what it was, and since most of management's recent communication had revolved around the implementation of cost-saving measures, everyone's assumption seemed to be that patient care was of secondary importance.

IT WASN'T GOOD ENOUGH TO "JUST" PROVIDE A GREAT IN-CLINIC EXPERIENCE. WE ALSO HAD TO PROVIDE GREAT SERVICE DURING EVERY POINT OF CONTACT WITH THE PATIENT BEFORE AND AFTER THE VISIT.

I began to fix this by introducing a new "Mission, Vision, and Values" for the company. I referenced these, in one way or another, in literally all my communications with team members, including lengthy monthly emails bringing everyone up to date on the company's progress. FastMed's new Mission was "To provide patients with the best end-to-end healthcare experience in terms of quality, accessibility, affordability and compassion." This carefully worded statement spoke for itself, but the "end-to-end" piece warranted particular attention because it was intended to draw every team member into our daily quest to fulfill the Mission. It wasn't good enough to "just" provide a great in-clinic experience. We also had to provide great service during every point of contact with the patient before and after the visit—from when they located one of our nearby clinics online to how we handled billing errors when they inevitably occurred.

The Values I introduced were Service, Teamwork, Accountability, and Transparency. Each Value had a very specific definition, but beyond that we broke down each Value into specific behaviors we wanted everyone to practice on a daily basis. For example, the definition of Transparency was "We are honest about our mistakes and the shortcomings of our systems and processes, so that we can continually improve as individuals and as a company." The way this Value was operationalized was as follows: (1) admit mistakes immediately; (2) when you identify problems, propose possible solutions; (3) ask for help when you need it; (4) share information, knowledge, and expertise; and (5) lean into tough conversations.

Transparency was a particularly important value for FastMed at the time because I wanted to encourage our team members to speak up without fear of retribution when mistakes were made or when systems or processes were not working the way they should or could. This way, we could fix what was broken and become the learning organization we needed to be. As in the case of our Mission, I reinforced FastMed's so-called STAT Values (an acronym for our four Values and med-speak for "urgent") at every opportunity. They also were displayed on everyone's screen saver, and we introduced a biweekly internal newsletter called "The STAT."

The third leg to the new strategy was to create a differentiated approach to service delivery, one that would ensure that FastMed consistently delivered the high levels of patient satisfaction that would result in repeat visits, referrals, and positive social media and Google reviews. I knew this would be even more critical to FastMed's growth than it was for RediClinic, because FastMed could not rely on the regular exposure to thousands of shoppers in its host retailers' stores to help drive patient volume.

I had read many books over the years on how to provide great customer service and had gotten good tips from many of them, but the one that resonated most to me was *Setting the Table* by famed New York City restauranteur, Danny Meyer.[9] Here's how I adapted his philosophy to FastMed in an email I sent to all team members a few months after I joined the company:

As we have discussed many times, providing great service is one of the keys to fulfilling our Mission, "To provide the best end-to-end healthcare experience in terms of quality, accessibility, affordability and compassion." In addition, Service is one of our core Values: "Our ultimate calling is to provide superior service to our patients, and to support our patient-facing team members in their quest to do this."

But what does great service really mean, and how do we truly differentiate ourselves in this area? That's the question I have been asking myself over the past few months, so I went on a quest to find out how other companies in other industries define and deliver great service.

Along the way, I came across a book by Danny Meyer, who is arguably the most successful restaurant executive in the country. If you've been to New York City, or even if you

---

9   Danny Meyer, *Setting the Table: The Transforming Power of Hospitality in Business* (New York: HarperCollins Publishers, 2006).

haven't, you may have heard of Union Square Café and Gramercy Tavern, which are consistently rated among the top restaurants in what may be the world's most competitive restaurant market. During the past 30 years, Meyer's Union Square Hospitality Group has opened these and more than fifteen other successful restaurants, and his Shake Shack chain is now a billion-dollar company. In another book I read recently called "The Culture Code: The Secrets of Highly Successful Groups," the author likened Gramercy Tavern's wait staff to the restaurant equivalent of a Navy SEAL team. In Meyer's book, "Setting the Table: The Transforming Power of Hospitality in Business," he attributes much of his company's success to their focus on hospitality, which is different from service in an important way. Here's how Meyer puts it:

> Service is the technical delivery of a product. Hospitality is how the delivery of that product makes its recipient feel. Service is a monologue—we decide how we want to do things and set our own standards for service. Hospitality is a dialogue. To be on a guest's side requires listening to that person with every sense, and following up with a thoughtful, appropriate, gracious response. It takes both great service and great hospitality to rise to the top.

This got me to thinking that we have an opportunity to adapt Meyer's philosophy to our business, and in the process set a new standard for service in the healthcare industry. I am calling it "Compassionate Hospitality" because healthcare is different from the restaurant business in that most of our customers come to us when they are not feeling well and thus need to be treated with compassion, as our mission states. Quite simply, our objective is to ensure that every patient feels better—physically and emotionally—after every FastMed visit. Again, from Meyer's book:

> Virtually nothing else is as important as how one is made to feel in any business transaction. Hospitality exists when you believe the other person is on your side ... Hospitality is present when something happens for you. It is absent when something happens to you. These two simple prepositions—for and to—express it all.[10]

In order to consistently deliver Compassionate Hospitality (using a football analogy), we need to play both good offense and good defense. Good offense requires that we set high service standards for every team member who interacts with patients in any capacity, and that we consistently meet them. Good defense means that we define the most effective service recovery techniques, AND empower all patient-facing team members to do whatever is necessary to ensure that patients give us another chance if they had a less than excellent experience the first time around. It will take some time to define these service and recovery standards, but we are in the process of doing this right now and plan to implement a Compassionate Hospitality training program by the end of this year.

---

10   Ibid.

Of course, Compassionate Hospitality begins at the front desk because this is generally the first human interaction our patients have with us. For this reason, and in recognition of the importance of this interaction and our team members who are responsible for it, we are changing the title of our Guest Service Specialists to Patient Service Advocates (new name/title badges are on the way). This title change is not just window dressing. It represents a fundamental shift in the way we want to interact with our patients. Here's how Meyer describes the difference. When he refers to agents, substitute advocates:

> In every business, there are employees who are the first point of contact with the customers (attendants at airport gates, receptionists at doctors' offices, bank tellers, executive assistants). These people can come across as agents or gatekeepers. An agent makes things happen for others. A gatekeeper sets up barriers to keep people out. We're looking for agents, and our staff members are responsible for monitoring their own performance. In that transaction, did I present myself as an agent or a gatekeeper. In the world of hospitality, there's rarely anything in between.

Knowing our patient-facing team members as I do, I am certain that we are already practicing Compassionate Hospitality at many of our clinics, but we need to practice it with every patient at every clinic, every day. It will take a lot of effort on everyone's part to achieve this goal, but when we do, we will be setting a new standard for customer service in healthcare, taking care of our patients in the way they deserve, and separating ourselves from our competitors in the process. I hope you agree with me that this is a worthy goal and look forward to working with all of you to achieve it.

Now with a new labor model in place, a cultural transformation underway, and a new service delivery philosophy, the turnaround strategy for FastMed had been defined. The next challenge was to assemble a management team that could execute it.

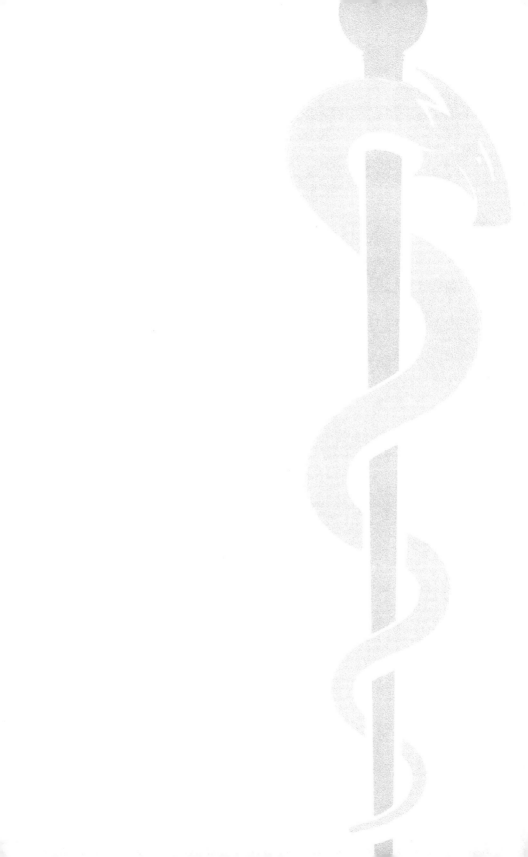

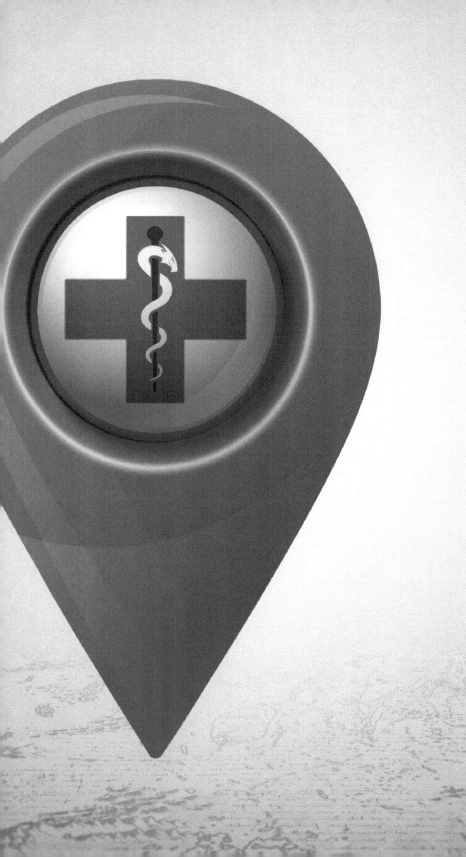

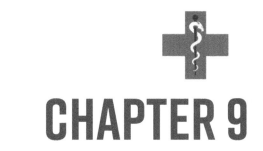

CHAPTER 9
BUILDING THE TEAM AND FACING THE GOVERNMENT

As previously mentioned, every member of FastMed's prior management team had resigned before my arrival at the company except their CFO. Kip respected him for his technical skills, and for having expressed his concerns about the company's direction before its troubles became obvious. However, while it was clear to me that he was a skilled and experienced financial executive, it was also apparent that he didn't share my passion for FastMed, my desire to transform it into a mission-driven enterprise, and my intention to ensure that the job of the corporate staff was to support our frontline team members. So, after a couple of months of trying to make the partnership work, we mutually agreed to part company.

This left me completely alone in the executive suite. Not that there weren't many good people at FastMed in our strange wedding venue offices in Gilbert, Arizona, and in our equally unusual corporate offices in Clayton, North Carolina, which were located across the road from the city dump. The first time I traveled there, the Uber driver's directions took us down City Dump Road, where he stopped in front of a large landfill and sheepishly turned around to ask me if this was really where I was intending to get out. Fortunately, it wasn't, but our real offices weren't exactly what I had in mind either, as they were inside a former supermarket distribution center with little shared space and lots of offices with closed doors and departmental sections that were walled off from each other. This was the antithesis of the open office configuration I favored and believed would be essential to getting everyone to start executing on our core value of Teamwork.

With FastMed's CFO now departed, I was relying on the director of finance for financial support, along with invaluable assistance from Kip, Nate Ott, Avery Zuck, and others at Abry Partners. This was a workable short-term solution, but I knew that it wasn't sustainable and that I desperately needed help in other functional areas as well. Fortunately, two ideal candidates soon emerged. I had wanted to bring RediClinic's talented CFO, Jeff Fields, with me to FastMed but assumed I couldn't because of a one-year non-solicitation clause in my Rite Aid separation agreement. However, Jeff became available earlier than I expected when he and Rite Aid mutually agreed to part company, so I snapped him up immediately.

At roughly the same time, I got an email from a former Blue Cross Blue Shield of North Carolina (BCBSNC) executive named Alex Gray expressing his interest in joining FastMed's leadership team. Alex had migrated to BCBSNC's venture arm, Echo Health Ventures, and in this capacity had served as a board advisor to FastMed, so he was familiar with the company. He also liked the new direction I was trying to take it and wanted to fill out his résumé with some operating experience. In addition, he had third-party payor experience, which I knew we would need. From his time at Echo, he was also familiar with the world of private equity. Best of all, he had an innovative, can-do spirit that was just what the FastMed doctor ordered. After a few meetings, Alex agreed to sign on as our chief growth officer.

The pieces of the leadership team were starting to fall into place, but the company still didn't have a chief operating officer. I had kept in touch with Danielle and wanted to try to convince her to join the FastMed team but couldn't yet because of my non-solicitation agreement. I could have tried to recruit someone else to fill that position but decided to hold out in hopes that Danielle would eventually become available. In the meantime, I reorganized the company into two regions—an Eastern Region that included all our clinics in North Carolina (roughly half of the company's total) and a Western Region that included our clinics in Arizona and Texas—and recruited a vice president of operations for each region.

In order to signal to all our team members that providing high-quality care was job #1, I elevated a senior physician in each region to the position of chief medical officer. One aspect of FastMed that had attracted me to the company was that it was the only independent urgent care operator in its three state markets that was Joint Commission accredited. Joint Commission accreditation is considered the gold standard of quality in the healthcare industry, and achieving it requires providers to survive a rigorous, time-consuming, and expensive inspection process, which is repeated every two years in order to maintain accreditation.

Most urgent care operators chose to forgo this process, relying mostly on the capabilities of their licensed providers. However, knowing that we had achieved Joint Commission accreditation helped me sleep better at night. I also believed that it gave us additional credibility with third-party payors and that maintaining accreditation would help us attract and retain the kinds of providers we would need to succeed in the future. That is, once we were able to give them the support they needed and deserved.

In addition to those I recruited from outside the company, there were many keepers from within FastMed as well. One was the company's vice president of marketing, Amrita Sahasrabudhe, whom Kip had recruited from PetSmart just prior to my arrival. I could see right away that she was very capable, committed to our new mission, and was exactly the right person to lead marketing and internal communications efforts. Another superstar was Christina Zeigler, who was the receptionist at FastMed's wedding venue offices and was the first person from the company I met on my first day. It didn't take me long to figure out that she was capable of doing a lot more than what she had been doing. She eventually turned out to be the best executive assistant to me and others and the best office manager and miscellaneous project manager I have ever had the pleasure of working with. There were others, too, who stepped up once they understood the company's new direction.

There were still management holes to fill, including chief technology officer, chief people officer, and general counsel, but we had enough horsepower to begin executing on our plan. FastMed's results began to improve almost immediately. The month-over-month visit volume declines were reversed, and the company began to generate profits at the unit level. Also, Net Promoter Scores were averaging more than 85, and clinic team member turnover had been cut in half. Enterprise profitability was still elusive because of the company's heavy debt load at near Mafia rates of 16–17 percent, but it was clear that FastMed was moving in the right direction, and Abry and other investors seemed pleased.

Then, in the summer of 2018, I received a call from Brent Stone—Abry's senior partner on their FastMed investment—informing me that they had reached a tentative agreement to acquire FastMed's largest competitor, NextCare, and wanted me and my team to run the combined company. FastMed and NextCare had been flirting with each other for years, as the logic of combining two of the largest urgent care companies was compelling. NextCare was slightly larger than FastMed, and most of their clinics were located in the same three states that we operated in. The combined company would be the largest urgent care and occupational health services operator in the nation, with sixty-seven clinics in North Carolina, seventy-three in Arizona, and sixty in Texas, and fifty-one clinics in seven other states.

The acquisition of NextCare would increase FastMed's profitability by enabling us to leverage our corporate overhead over a much larger footprint while creating millions of dollars of synergies through the elimination of overlapping corporate functions. It would also help solve a couple of state-specific problems I had begun to grapple with. With only twenty-one clinics in Texas, for example, FastMed didn't have enough scale and density in key regional markets to create operational and marketing efficiency. And, in Arizona, unfavorable reimbursement rates in our legacy payor contracts put a low ceiling on our potential profitability. Combining with NextCare would enable us to piggyback on their more favorable payor contracts in Arizona, and adding their thirty-nine clinics in Texas would solve our subscale problem there. I was less enthusiastic about NextCare's smaller positions in states other than Texas, Arizona, and North Carolina, but I figured we could either bulk up in those states post-close or sell NextCare's clinics in those states to reduce the net acquisition cost.

All in all, it was pretty darned exciting! At the end of 2018, we signed a definitive agreement to purchase NextCare, began the integration process, and submitted information about the transaction to the Federal Trade Commission (FTC) as required under Hart-Scott-Rodino because the size of the transaction was over the legal threshold. At the time, it never occurred to me—or to anyone else involved with either company—that the FTC would take exception to the planned merger of FastMed and NextCare or even notice it for that matter. They had recently approved the acquisition of Time Warner by AT&T, and it looked like they were going to green-light the acquisition of Sprint by T-Mobile (which they eventually did), so how could they possibly care about the relatively small and inconsequential transaction between FastMed and NextCare? Well, we would find out one way or the other within thirty days of our filing, as required by law.

We had one unusual thing going against us that could not have been anticipated, which was the government shutdown at the end of 2018 caused by the failure of the Administration and Congress to agree on an increase in the debt ceiling. This meant that there were very few employees working at the FTC to review our filing when it was submitted in late December, which impaired their ability to evaluate the transaction within the statutory thirty-day period. I'll never know what really happened behind the scenes at the FTC, but in any case, we were both surprised and distressed to receive their dreaded second request for information at the end of January 2019 in the form of a forty-page, single-spaced document that solicited information on every conceivable aspect of both companies' businesses—past, present, and planned future.

While we and our lawyers were incredibly disappointed, we remained confident that rationality would prevail within the FTC and set about responding to their information request while proceeding with integration planning. By this time, my non-solicitation period had ended, and I immediately contacted Danielle in an effort to convince her to join the FastMed team as chief operating officer. Rite Aid had continued to have challenges, most recently in the form of a failed merger with Albertsons and John Standley's subsequent departure from the company, so Danielle was ready for a change. She was looking to return to a more entrepreneurial environment, as I had been, and fortunately was willing to join forces with me once again.

As we began to dig into the FTC's concerns, it was apparent that they believed our increased scale in North Carolina, Arizona, and Texas would lead to an increase in the cost of healthcare in these three states due to the increased leverage they thought we would have over the payors in those states. This was preposterous on its face because even with our increased number of clinics, FastMed would still have a very small market share for the limited services we offered and very little ability to command increased reimbursement rates. Payors had other types of providers in their networks that offered similar services, including physician practices with open hours, hospital emergency rooms, a growing number of retail-based clinics (I had created a monster!), and emerging telemedicine providers.

However, the FTC stubbornly refused to acknowledge that FastMed was not just competing against other urgent care providers and insisted upon defining our market shares by calculating the number of urgent care clinics the combined FastMed-NextCare would have in its three core states as a percentage of the total number of urgent care clinics in those states and the key markets within them. The irrationality of this was very frustrating, and equally unsettling was the amount of resources the FTC was dedicating to this relatively small transaction. In addition to all the information from us and other sources they had requested and were reviewing, we had three in-person meetings with the FTC at their headquarters in Washington, DC, in which they were represented by at least six staff lawyers and economists. They were always polite and agreeable in our meetings, but it was difficult to know whether we were making any headway, and the whole process struck me—with my citizen hat on—as a colossal waste of taxpayer resources.

THE FUNDAMENTAL PROBLEM WAS THAT WE WERE ON A CLOCK AND A BUDGET, WHILE THE FTC WAS NOT.

The fundamental problem was that we were on a clock and a budget, while the FTC was not. Huge companies like AT&T and Time Warner expect to take months, if not years, to secure regulatory approval for their multi-billion-dollar mergers and can afford to spend many millions of dollars in legal fees to do it. Conversely, FastMed had a limited budget for legal expenses and commitments from lenders that were necessary to finance the acquisition were scheduled to terminate in April. With more time and money, I believed we eventually would have secured FTC approval, perhaps contingent upon divesting some of NextCare's clinics in markets where the combined companies would have more than 30 percent market share according to the FTC's narrow definition. However, we were rapidly running out of time, and the uncertainty over whether the two companies were merging or not was weighing heavily on both organizations.

In the end, we agreed with NextCare to call off the merger rather than continue to subject both companies to an expensive and seemingly endless regulatory process with an uncertain outcome.

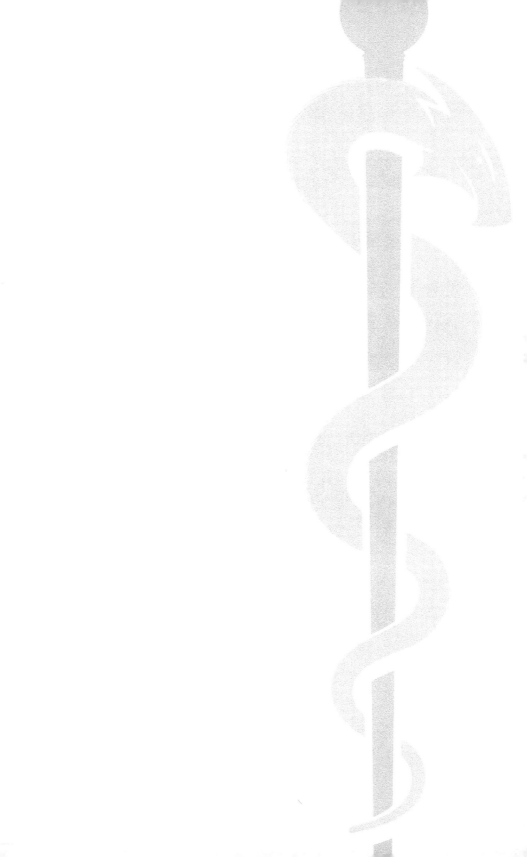

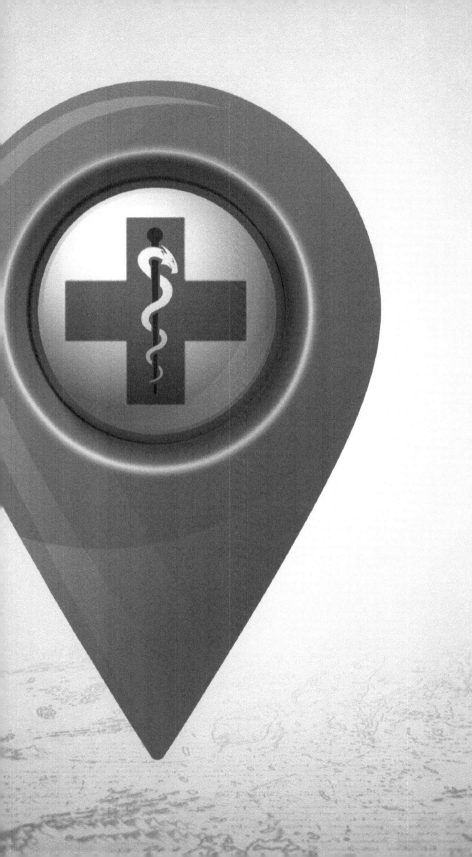

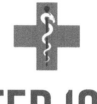

CHAPTER 10
OUT OF THE FRYING PAN AND
INTO THE PANDEMIC FIRE

The collapse of FastMed's acquisition of NextCare left us in a very precarious position. While FastMed's financial results had improved significantly since I had joined the company about a year and a half before, we were still struggling with the high-priced debt I had inherited, whose interest payments increasingly had to be paid in cash rather than in shares. Abry had counted on the lower cost debt we had planned to raise through Barclays to not only finance the acquisition but also take out our current high-cost lender, BlueMountain Capital. Abry also counted on the synergies to be gained from the acquisition and on NextCare's accretive profits to minimize the need for additional equity investments.

When none of these things occurred, the principals at Abry told me that they could no longer support the company. This was a blow financially but an even heavier one because Kip, Brent, Nate, Avery, and others from Abry had been incredibly supportive operationally and in other nonfinancial ways. I knew we were going to miss them, but they understood the precariousness of our position—and to their everlasting credit—offered to relinquish most of their equity to new investors if we could find any. In addition, they connected us with excellent restructuring counsel at Kirkland & Ellis and investment bankers at Houlihan Lokey.

Fortunately, we had two viable restructuring options that would allow us to avoid bankruptcy. One option was that FastMed's other main investors, Falcon Investment Advisors and Blue Cross Blue Shield of North Carolina (BCBSNC)—through their venture arm, Echo Health Ventures—were interested in making add-on equity investments in a restructured FastMed. They also brought in a well-regarded private equity firm, Crestline Investors, to replace BlueMountain's expensive debt with a loan on more favorable terms and make an equity investment alongside Falcon and BCBSNC. The second option was that BlueMountain was interested in acquiring a control position in FastMed, by converting some of their high-priced debt into equity and making a new equity investment.

To secure investments from the groups led by Falcon or Blue-Mountain, we had to prepare a multi-year business plan that would give both groups the confidence to proceed. In addition to continuing with the three near-term strategies we had laid out—to implement a more flexible and data-driven clinic staffing model, foster a mission- and values-driven culture, and adopt the "Compassionate Hospitality" service delivery model—we defined three longer-term strategies:

1. Become an omnichannel provider, with the goal of being able to treat patients virtually if their conditions allowed for it. If not, they would be referred to one of our nearby clinics.

2. Add family medicine to our urgent care and occupational health service lines in a growing number of clinics. We already had successfully piloted this concept in five so-called hybrid clinics in North Carolina, based on research showing that more than 40 percent of our urgent care patients said they did not have a primary care provider and would strongly consider using FastMed for many primary care needs if we offered these services.

3. Expand our presence in key Texas markets to increase marketing and operational efficiency and lift our reimbursement rates in Arizona through renegotiation of our payor contracts or other means.

With our new five-year plan in hand, we had multiple conversations with the Falcon-led investor group and with BlueMountain, and both continued to be interested. I favored the Falcon group for several reasons: they had been consistently supportive in the past; I had developed strong personal relationships with principals at both Falcon and BCBSNC/Echo; and my initial impressions of Crestline, which was based in my home state of Texas, had been positive. In addition, one of the principals at BlueMountain had been overly aggressive in challenging management during one of our presentations, and I suspected that this was the way it might be if we buckled up with them.

To be clear, it wasn't the fact that we were challenged, as I have always welcomed the opinions of others as a means of getting to the best solution. However, the tone of the challenge in this instance was disrespectful, which is something I have very little tolerance for. As it turned out, BlueMountain seemed happy to have us repay their high-priced loan at a considerable profit when we ultimately opted to move forward with the Falcon-led group.

With FastMed now officially "restructured," and with fresh capital in the bank, we proceeded enthusiastically to begin implementing our plan. To operationalize our strategy to become an omnichannel provider and move into family medicine, I felt strongly that FastMed needed to convert to a new electronic health record (EHR) system. EHRs are the backbone of most providers' businesses, as they are essential to both patient care and revenue cycle management.

However, the EHR FastMed was using when I joined the company had fallen behind the technology curve and did not support virtual care. It also was difficult to extract the kinds of data from the outdated system that we would need to assess our performance against quality benchmarks and assume risk in an environment where third-party payors were moving to contracts based on the "value" of the care provided, rather than on the volume of visits, tests, and procedures.

We cast a wide net in search of a new EHR, carefully assessing the functionality, cost, and strategic advantages of each one of the leading systems. After an extensive review, we concluded that Epic would be our best choice from a functionality and strategic standpoint. We could utilize its native telemedicine capability, benefit from the "stickiness" of its industry leading "MyChart" patient portal, and gain easy access to large datasets. Also, converting to Epic would enable us to clinically integrate with the many large health systems in our markets that used the market-leading system or were in the process of converting to it. In addition, we were impressed with Epic's team and believed they had the resources and disposition to be a good technology partner.

The two main negatives were that Epic had a high up-front cost and that FastMed would be the first independent urgent care operator to implement a system that—while generally considered to be best-in-class—had been primarily designed for large health systems. With respect to cost, our analysis showed that Epic's high up-front cost relative to other systems would be counterbalanced by a lower cost of ownership over the five-year duration of our new plan. And while we were justifiably nervous about the prospect of being the first in our urgent care niche to convert to Epic, we felt that being an innovator was in our DNA, and we were confident that the detailed implementation plan Epic had prepared for us would work.

Major EHR system conversions are always challenging, partially due to the need for extensive retraining of providers and front-desk and back-office personnel. Conversions to Epic, even among large health systems with far greater resources than FastMed, had occasionally gone awry, so we knew it was going to be a heavy lift and prepared accordingly by positioning it as a "Moon Shot" within our organization. As it turned out, the launch meeting we had in Raleigh, in February 2020, for more than one hundred team members who were to be heavily involved in the Epic Moon Shot was the last large in-person meeting we would have until COVID-19 began to subside two years later.

While we continued to run virtual care pilots and refine our hybrid clinic model, the Epic conversion was a gating item for the full implementation of each initiative. Therefore, at the beginning of 2020, we concentrated mainly on preparing for the conversion and on other aspects of our plan that were not dependent on the new system. One important objective was to increase our payor reimbursement rates in Arizona, which were below market and limited our profitability in the state even though our patient volumes had increased significantly during the previous two years. Alex and I had tried to renegotiate with payors directly, but I was skeptical about whether we would be successful in a time frame that was consistent with our plan's financial projections.

Prior to our decision to pursue the acquisition of NextCare, I had engaged with executives at a leading health system in Arizona called HonorHealth about the possibility of forming a joint venture (JV). This would raise cash for FastMed through the sale of a 51 percent stake in our Arizona clinics and, in the process, enable the JV to piggyback on the higher reimbursement rates that large health systems like Honor usually were able to command. The principal executive at HonorHealth I had worked with on the JV had been justifiably disappointed when I had told him in late 2018 that the deal had to be back-burnered due to our refocus on the NextCare acquisition. So, I was pleasantly surprised when he called following the announcement in April 2019 that FastMed's acquisition of NextCare would not occur to ask if we wanted to restart JV discussions between our two organizations.

The logic of the JV was no less compelling for both parties at that point than it had been prior to the NextCare diversion. FastMed needed cash for expansion, higher reimbursement rates, and upstream referrals. And Honor needed an expanded community presence, downstream referrals, and a partner that understood retail medicine. In addition, Honor had recently converted to Epic and FastMed was about to, so the partnership would realize the benefits of true clinical integration—including seamless patient medical record sharing—that rarely existed in the nation's balkanized healthcare delivery system. As 2020 began, we were focused strategically on preparing for our conversion to the new Epic system and finalizing our JV with HonorHealth. And then, of course, everything changed.

Patient volumes in January and the first part of February 2020 were significantly ahead of budget, and then, in March, COVID-19 hit us like a ton of bricks. Patient volumes immediately fell by more than 50 percent as a result of government-mandated shutdowns. In addition, our clinic team members were understandably concerned about their jobs and safety, and some of the Personal Protective Equipment (PPE) we needed to keep them safe was impossible to secure at reasonable prices, if at all. As it became clear that FastMed was on the front lines of a global pandemic whose severity and duration were uncertain, the plan we had carefully developed would have to be tabled and replaced with one better suited to the crisis we were now facing.

Working closely with other members of our leadership team, I created a new plan called "Operation Resilience" that was shared with more than 1,000 FastMed team members in a video town hall at the end of April 2020. It had five guiding principles:

- Stay true to FastMed's Mission and Values.
- Take care of our team members, particularly with respect to their safety and job security.
- Manage cash closely (think like a start-up, and prepare forecasts based on conservative assumptions).
- Share the pain with key partners, to reduce near-term costs wherever possible.
- Keep the long-term plan intact (think in two time zones).

The philosophy and approach we described in the town hall had four key elements:

- We're all in this together.
- Combine brutal honesty with a rational basis for hope. To underscore this point, I quoted from Adm. James Stockdale who had been captured by the Vietcong and brutally tortured during more than seven years in the Hanoi Hilton: "You must never confuse faith that you will prevail—which you can never afford to lose—with the discipline to confront the most brutal facts of your reality, whatever they may be."
- Focus on what we can control.
- Overcommunicate (share information, invite engagement, respond appreciatively).

I also emphasized that we needed to be agile:

- Identify and understand evolving and emerging issues. (What do we know and *not* know, and what are the implications for our current [default] plan?)
- Develop options.
- Predict outcomes for each option.
- Choose the best course of action.
- Execution-as-learning.

I then introduced three key components of our new plan:

- Accelerate the deployment of telemedicine/virtual care (which was launching in all states that week).
- Introduce and expand our array of COVID testing options and locations.
- Implement what I referred to as "Smart Clinic Management," in which we would strive to keep all clinics open

and all full-time team members employed but would need to reduce hours of operation at some clinics and would work with the affected team members to offset pay reductions through the use of paid-time-off (PTO) balances and unemployment insurance.

I went on to discuss some of the implications of COVID-19 for FastMed, stressing that while patient volumes would be depressed in the short term, FastMed's strategic plan to implement a high-quality, accessible, and afford-able physical/virtual care delivery model to serve as the "front door" to healthcare would make perfect sense in a post-COVID world, as well as during it. I ended with the famous quote from Andy Grove, former CEO of Intel, which I never tire of remembering and wholeheartedly believe: "Bad companies are destroyed by crisis, Good companies survive them, Great companies are improved by them."

The approach, key messages, and plans of Operation Resilience seemed to resonate with team members, although everyone knew FastMed was in a tough spot. As it turned out, patient volumes increased as the mandated shutdowns were gradually lifted, and we made it through the pandemic without having to furlough any full-time team members.

However, it was a very difficult time, particularly for our patient-facing team members, because sometimes they had no patients at all and at other times were overwhelmed by more than they could handle (FastMed managed 2.4 million mostly COVID-related patient visits in 2021 alone). In addition, many patients were difficult to deal with duc to their understandable frustration over long lines and their fear of the unknown, while our team members who treated them were uncomfortable in their masks, shields, and gloves, sometimes sick themselves and increasingly worn down by the daily stress of it all. I had tremendous respect for their resilience, and we began referring to them as the "Healthcare Heroes" I sincerely believe they are.

Despite the massive immediate challenges of being on the front lines of a pandemic, and in order to honor our commitment to "think in two time zones," we needed to press forward on our two key strategic initiatives for the year. Our negotiations with Honor continued to progress even though both provider organizations were stressed by COVID-19, and the JV was formed in August. Meanwhile, we had decided to implement Epic on a rolling, state-specific basis beginning with Arizona in the fourth quarter because of the opportunity to clinically integrate with Honor via our respective instances of the same EHR.

The Epic implementation would have been a heavy lift under normal circumstances, but the pandemic made it an even heavier one because the extensive team member training on the new system had to be done virtually. Nevertheless, implementations in Arizona— and subsequently in Texas and North Carolina during the first half of 2021—were reasonably successful, though there were issues both at the point of care and in the processing of claims that increased the level of team member frustration and negatively impacted our short-term cash flow. I knew from discussions with other healthcare providers who had converted to Epic that these issues would occur, but they were particularly difficult to deal with in the context of our already challenging pandemic environment.

As if the combination of our Epic conversion and COVID-19 were not enough, I was considering adding a third piece to the disruptive puzzle that had the potential to stress our organization to the breaking point and also could vault FastMed into an undisputed leadership position in the urgent care business. Here be Dragons!

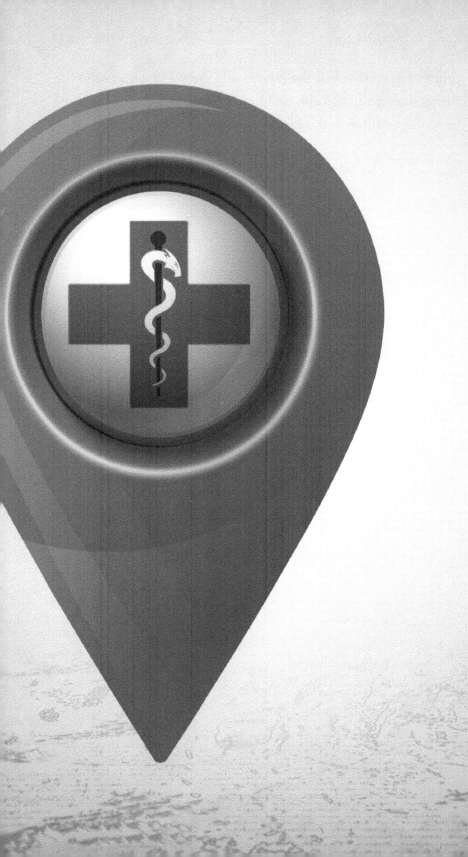

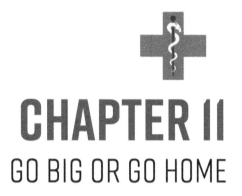

CHAPTER 11
GO BIG OR GO HOME

Since one of our business plan goals was to increase FastMed's scale in key Texas markets, I had contacted an investment banker named Gordon Maner who was a principal at a boutique firm called AMB and asked him to keep his eyes out for tuck-in acquisition opportunities in Houston, Austin, and San Antonio. I also suggested we would be interested in tuck-in opportunities in Arizona and North Carolina and even in entering a new state if it was growing rapidly like our current state markets and we could achieve significant scale in a single transaction. I had known Gordon for many years, as he was one of the first investment bankers to see potential in the emerging retail medicine sector, and I admired the energy and deal-making skill he and his team brought to it.

One day in early 2020—shortly after the pandemic had begun to upend our business—Gordon called to say he had heard that Tenet Healthcare, the nation's second largest publicly traded healthcare provider, was interested in selling its large stable of urgent care clinics that operated under the MedPost brand in Texas, Arizona, and California and under the CareSpot brand in Florida. Coincidentally, CareSpot's predecessor company, Solantic, had been founded by Rick Scott and had to be sold when he became governor of Florida due to potential conflicts of interest. Before the divestiture occurred, Rick and I had discussed the possibility of combining RediClinic and Solantic, and I had visited the Solantic clinics at that time and been impressed by them.

I was interested in pursuing the Tenet opportunity because their clinics would enable us to bulk up in Texas and Arizona and enter the high-growth state of Florida in a meaningful way. We quickly engaged AMB to represent us, and they threw our hat into the ring. It turned out that other bidders were ahead of us, but we had a chance if we could move quickly. Upon closer inspection, we found that Tenet owned twenty-one MedPost clinics in Texas, which would enable us to roughly double our presence in key markets there. They also owned six MedPost clinics in the Phoenix area, which would add to our JV's market presence in Arizona, as well as seventeen MedPost clinics in Southern California. In Florida, they operated forty-three CareSpot clinics, most of which were jointly owned with four leading health systems, a model I had used successfully at RediClinic and more recently at FastMed with HonorHealth in Arizona.

The intelligence we got through AMB was that many of the other bidders were lusting after Florida, as the CareSpot clinics were located not only in one of the nation's fastest growing states but also in many of its fastest growing markets—including Jacksonville and Orlando.

However, we also learned that Tenet wanted to sell their urgent care clinics in all four states in a single transaction, and they wanted to be certain that the buyer had the ability to close (no financing risk) and could close quickly.

The fact that Tenet wanted to sell all their clinics to a single buyer played into our hands because none of the other parties that were interested in the Florida clinics—to our knowledge—already operated clinics in Texas and Arizona, and thus, they could not partially justify a purchase price based on the strategic value of increased density in the latter two states the way we could. I was less enthusiastic about acquiring Tenet's California clinics due to the state's difficult regulatory environment, and because their seventeen MedPost clinics lacked sufficient density, but I thought we would be able to sell these clinics to another buyer after the acquisition if we decided not to stay the course there.

On the other hand, purchasing all eighty-seven of Tenet's clinics was a much larger transaction than our company and its investors had been prepared to support. Nevertheless, all of us could see that acquiring Tenet's clinics would make FastMed one of the nation's largest urgent care and occupational health services operators, with strong positions in four of the nation's fastest growing states and many of the fastest growing markets within them. This seemed like a once-in-a-business-lifetime opportunity.

After much internal discussion and several rounds of negotiation with Tenet, we agreed on a purchase price and executed a nonbinding letter of intent in August 2020. We then proceeded to pull the necessary funds together, combining proceeds from the sale of our 51 percent stake to HonorHealth with additional commitment from each of our current shareholders. With this financing in place, we signed a definitive agreement with Tenet in December 2020 and announced that the transaction was expected to close during the first half of the following year.

Remembering that we had signed a definitive purchase agreement with NextCare two years earlier, in December 2018, and had been tripped up by the FTC in the first half of the following year, I wondered what could possibly foil us this time, as the Tenet transaction was not reportable under Hart-Scott-Rodino because the purchase price was below the then-current threshold.

We were scheduled to close at the end of February 2021, just as the Omicron variant of COVID was surging and continuing to disrupt both FastMed's and Tenet's urgent care businesses. While this gave us pause, we also had not yet satisfied two Florida-related closing conditions that were baked into the purchase agreement for our protection. The first was that we had not been able to secure a sufficient number of FastMed contracts with third-party payors in Florida, as the CareSpot clinics would no longer be able to piggyback on Tenet's national payor contracts. The second was that some of the state-required clinic license transfers had not been completed.

Our purchase agreement with Tenet allowed for an extension of the closing date to enable these two workstreams to be completed but only upon mutual agreement of the parties. Tenet was initially unwilling to grant the extension, partly because they had counted on a speedy close, and because they may have thought we were vacillating due to COVID-related market uncertainties, but they finally agreed to a sixty-day extension in connection with a breakup fee if we didn't meet the new deadline.

The breakup fee wasn't so large that we couldn't have backed out of the deal, but the investment thesis for the transaction remained sound: the price was attractive, the potential synergies to be achieved through the business combination were substantial, and the strategic benefits were undeniable. So, our board elected to proceed with the acquisition despite the impact of COVID, provided we were able to meet the payor contract transfer goal and complete all the license transfers before the sixty-day extension ran out.

This was a great example of "thinking in two time zones," as we had committed ourselves to do in Operation Resilience. Still, I knew that integrating an acquisition that would nearly double FastMed's size would push the envelope operationally, especially in the middle of a pandemic and following closely on the heels of a complex EHR conversion.

Companies that make acquisitions in similar businesses tend to approach their acquisitions in one of two ways: either they essentially force their people, systems, and processes onto the acquired company in the belief that they know best how everything should be run and who should run it, or they try to identify and implement the best people, systems, and processes from both organizations. The former approach has the advantage of clarity and speed but may not produce the best long-term results. The latter approach takes more time and tends to create near-term uncertainty in both organizations, but it can produce superior long-term results. I opted for this approach, believing that we had the time and respecting the fact that CareSpot|MedPost (CSMP) had been an urgent care pioneer, just like FastMed. In addition, I had been impressed by many of CSMP's people and by some of their systems and processes during our due

> I KNEW THAT INTEGRATING AN ACQUISITION THAT WOULD NEARLY DOUBLE FASTMED'S SIZE WOULD PUSH THE ENVELOPE OPERATIONALLY, ESPECIALLY IN THE MIDDLE OF A PANDEMIC AND FOLLOWING CLOSELY ON THE HEELS OF A COMPLEX EHR CONVERSION.

diligence process and was excited about incorporating them into an enhanced FastMed operating model.

To make it clear to everyone that we were going to be thoughtful and open-minded throughout the integration process, and to facilitate the combination of the two organizations, I instinctively felt that it would be helpful to include a member of CSMP's executive team on FastMed's go-forward executive team. During the diligence process, I had been particularly impressed with their chief financial officer (CFO), Dan Murphy, who had been with CSMP for more than a decade and had assembled a strong finance and accounting team that seemed to be firing on all cylinders. After much deliberation and discussion with other members of our board, I decided that we should appoint Dan as FastMed's new CFO. This was a very difficult decision because it meant that we would have to part ways with Jeff Fields, who I had worked closely with at both RediClinic and FastMed—and who I both liked and respected—but I believed that it was the right decision for the company at this delicate point in its evolution.

Dan and his team were immediately faced with a host of financial issues that had multiple causes. While we had scraped together enough money to complete the CSMP acquisition, FastMed didn't have much cash in the bank afterward despite having put an asset-based line of credit in place. More importantly, our ability to generate cash from operations was severely hampered by pandemic-related rising labor costs and staffing shortages and by the ongoing denials of claims that were submitted through our new Epic system. There were also delays in receiving reimbursements under new payor contracts, including those from Honor, and even under some existing payor contracts where tax identification numbers had to be changed because of the acquisition.

Moreover, having essentially completed the conversion to Epic in the legacy FastMed clinics, we were now back to managing two EHRs because CSMP used another system called NextGen. The plan was to convert all clinics to Epic, but this would be an expensive and time-consuming process that was slowed by our reluctance to continue rolling out a new system before the revenue cycle issues had been resolved, as well as by the cash crunch that the company as a whole was experiencing.

The problem of having two EHR systems was especially acute in Texas, where half of our clinics were on Epic and the other half on NextGen, and where marketing efficiency was constrained by the fact that we were also operating under two different brands. All of these issues had been predicted, and I knew it could be resolved over time, but it was painful in the interim for all FastMed team members and shareholders alike.

Nevertheless, the integration was progressing relatively smoothly, and there were some pieces of good news. One was that before the end of the year we were able to sell our seventeen MedPost clinics in California to Carbon Health—an emerging company that already had a substantial presence in the state—for an amount that covered a significant portion of what we had paid Tenet for all eighty-seven clinics. This validated our belief that we had made a good deal in purchasing CSMP. Ironically, however, the combination of this successful transaction and the operational challenges we were facing caused our board to start thinking about whether we should consider selling FastMed, either as a whole or in pieces. I was against doing this because I believed that we would realize far more value for FastMed if we were given time to execute on our five-year plan, but I also understood why the shareholders—including me—would be tempted by the opportunity to monetize our investments that the Carbon transaction suggested was possible.

As of this writing, it appears that FastMed will be sold. I am sad about this because we were in the process of building a great company that has already provided high-quality, accessible, and affordable healthcare to patients representing nearly ten million visits, and the planned enhancements to our model of care would have enabled us to serve more patients in even more valuable ways. Whether this happens at FastMed or at other companies, there is still much work to be done to make our nation's healthcare system more responsive and sustainable. What I know now after spending the past thirty-five years trying to achieve this goal is that it is tremendously challenging but that it is possible if you have the creativity, determination, and team to do it.

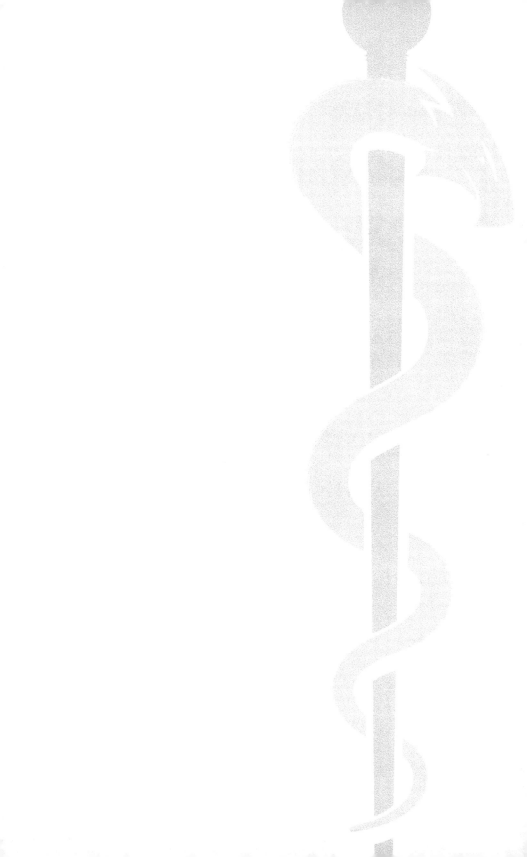

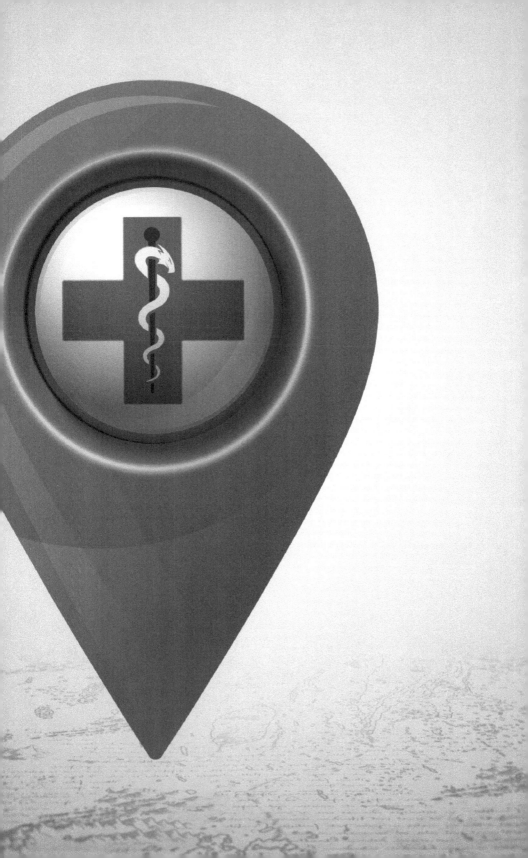

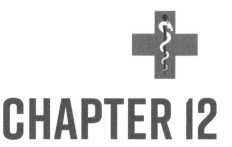

CHAPTER 12
LEADERSHIP ON THE RAZOR'S EDGE

My efforts over the past thirty-five years to make reliable health information and care more accessible have been rewarding but challenging. Thanks to the talent and dedication of many teammates, I believe we have had a positive impact on our nation's inefficient healthcare delivery system, but our progress has been hard fought and certainly not in a straight line. More like three yards and a cloud of dust!

Nevertheless, I have learned a few things along the way about leading during times that have become increasingly unpredictable in a general sense and about leading companies that are trying to break the mold without knowing exactly what the new one should look like. I don't claim that any of these leadership lessons are original, but I can attest to the fact that they are battle-tested and worked for me.

The first and most important thing I have found about leadership—particularly in healthcare—is that to be effective, you have to be as passionate about the mission as you are about the financial results. I was fortunate to have found my passion in healthcare, and my mission to make it more accessible and affordable is what has kept me going through thick and thin and what has enabled me to attract such great people to join in this quest. Not that financial results are unimportant, because as we used to say at RediClinic, "No Money, No Mission!" However, most of the individuals a healthcare provider organization will need to be successful are primarily (and fortunately) motivated by the desire to improve the health and well-being of their patients, and you will not be able to attract and retain the best of these patient-facing team members if they think it's all about the money.

> **THE FIRST AND MOST IMPORTANT THING I HAVE FOUND ABOUT LEADERSHIP—PARTICULARLY IN HEALTHCARE—IS THAT TO BE EFFECTIVE, YOU HAVE TO BE AS PASSIONATE ABOUT THE MISSION AS YOU ARE ABOUT THE FINANCIAL RESULTS.**

My second key leadership tenet is that your #1 job should be to find good people and help them grow. No matter how talented and committed you are, you will not achieve anything of consequence if you aren't able to surround yourself with individuals who are equally if not more capable in certain areas and ways than you are. Sometimes these individuals already exist inside or outside of your organization, but frequently, you have to find people who have potential and mentor them. This usually means that you have to let them fail from time to time rather than constantly jumping in to do their jobs for them when you think they might be falling short. This is hard for type-As like me to accept, but you have to do it, or your company will never have the human capital it needs to grow beyond your own limited ceiling.

In order to attract and retain these kinds of individuals, you have to learn how to serve them. Much has been written about the concept of "servant leadership," so I won't repeat it here, but I can say without reservation that it works. If people know you are there to support them and have their backs—as long as they are honest and hard-working—this will create the kind of discretionary effort that is required for companies to succeed against all odds. I'm not saying that you don't need to define the vision, drive for results, or make the tough calls, but your main job is to set aggressive but

> **NO MATTER HOW TALENTED AND COMMITTED YOU ARE, YOU WILL NOT ACHIEVE ANYTHING OF CONSEQUENCE IF YOU AREN'T ABLE TO SURROUND YOURSELF WITH INDIVIDUALS WHO ARE EQUALLY IF NOT MORE CAPABLE IN CERTAIN AREAS AND WAYS THAN YOU ARE.**

realistic goals, make sure your direct reports have the resources they need to achieve them, and then monitor their efforts and progress in a supportive manner.

Part of this is making sure they (and others in the organization) get most of the credit for goal achievement, even if you played an important part in making it happen. Someone once said that there is no limit to what you can accomplish if you don't care who gets the credit, and I have generally found this to be true. Money is always important, but for many people, recognition is equally, if not more, important, so you need to take advantage of every opportunity to provide it.

Conversely, you need to ultimately own whatever didn't work or isn't working. Jocko Willink and Leif Babin elaborate on this concept very effectively in their book, *Extreme Ownership*, and I totally subscribe to it.[11] If you want to be an effective leader, you must give most of the credit to others and take all the blame for yourself. If your ego is too big and fragile to handle this, then your chances of success will be significantly diminished.

Since things will frequently not go as planned, particularly in early-stage companies for which there is no proven business model, good leaders must learn to embrace all obstacles. Ryan Holiday describes this very well in his book, *The Obstacle Is the Way*, in which he stresses the importance of seeing every obstacle as an opportunity for improvement.[12]

Long gone are the days when leaders could simply "plan the work and work the plan." As Mike Tyson famously said, "Everyone has a plan before they get punched in the mouth." Good leaders expect to be punched in the mouth on a regular basis and, rather than letting it get them down, use it as fuel to take their businesses to the next level. Success is frequently not a matter of what happens to you and your company but how you react to the inevitable twists and turns along the way. This is much easier said than done, but I have found that it is possible if you take a page out of Stoicism (read especially the works of Marcus Aurelius and Seneca) and always focus on what you can control.

It is also important to remember that, as Billy Jean King said, "Pressure is a privilege." When you're feeling sorry for yourself because it seems like the weight of the world is on your shoulders, it helps to remember that it is a privilege and a responsibility to others that you are in a position to make a difference.

---

11   Jocko Willink and Leif Babin, *Summary of Extreme Ownership, by Jocko Willink and Leif Babin* (2019) Author's Republic.

12   Ryan Holiday, *The Obstacle Is the Way: The Timeless Art of Turning Trials Into Triumph* (New York: Portfolio/Penguin, 2014).

The daunting challenges of running any business in these turbulent times can put tremendous personal pressure on leaders and tempt them to take shortcuts—financially and in ways they interact with others—but good leaders don't succumb to these temptations. As General Norman Schwarzkopf once said, "The truth of the matter is that you always know the right thing to do. The hard part is doing it." It's a simple statement but one that I have found to be remarkably accurate. I can't remember a single ethical dilemma I have faced over the years when I didn't know in my heart how I should handle it.

Fortunately, I had parents and other role models who stressed the importance of truth telling and personal integrity, but sometimes it's very difficult to do the right thing even when you know what it is. This is particularly the case when you are under the most pressure because things have not worked out the way you expected or hoped they would. Don't ever give into the temptation to cut corners. Your career (and your life) is a marathon—not a 100-yard dash—and your reputation can either help you or hurt you at every step along the way.

Good leaders are known not only for their integrity but also for their work ethic. It seems obvious, but I have always found that you have to work extra hard to accomplish anything of consequence, and you have to be incredibly persistent and have a tendency to never take "no" for an answer.

I ran across an interview many years ago with one of the few fellow Harvard graduates who was playing in the NFL. Harvard doesn't give athletic scholarships, so it doesn't necessarily attract the nation's best athletes, but this guy appeared to have become a reasonably successful, if undersized, linebacker. When the interviewer asked him how he had made it in the NFL despite not having the college pedigree and physical attributes of a typical professional football player, he responded that he had a sign in his bedroom that read, "Let no one outwork you today." Hard work is how you beat the odds and set the right example for your teammates.

With that said, you're not going to be a good leader if you are so focused on your job that it negatively impacts your health and family relationships. You must have an outlet that enables you to blow off steam in a positive way, and for me that has always been exercise. I have been accused of taking it to an extreme, but even at my relatively advanced age, I generally get at least two hours of vigorous exercise every day, almost always in the very early morning before the workday begins and (in the old days) before my family was awake.

I've been a longtime runner (including marathons) because it's the easiest form of exercise to do when traveling, but I mix it up with lifting, rowing, swimming, tennis, golf (always walk and carry my bag), and fitness routines that one of my sons taught me from his time in the Marine Corps. The benefits of exercise for me have always been as much mental as physical, as exercise has allowed me to disconnect from my phone and computer and think more clearly than I am frequently able to in the middle of a busy day. In addition, exercise has helped me sleep better at night knowing that I will have uninterrupted time before going to work the following morning to reflect on whatever pressing matters need to be resolved.

Another important aspect of work-life balance is staying in touch with your family and nonwork friends. This is not easy when you are pulling eighty-hour workweeks, constantly stressed and distracted by work-related challenges, and spending most of your time with co-workers. The danger here is not only that you have little time and energy left over for anyone else but also that being in the bunker with co-workers can strengthen these relationships to the point that they may seem more important than any others.

While I have been fortunate to have made many lifelong friends through work, my family members and nonwork friends have provided a combination of dependable sustenance, pride and joy, healthy distraction, and a sense of purpose that was not available elsewhere. However, this does not happen if you don't consciously nurture nonwork relationships, so you must make time and be present for them.

Finally, you cannot allow yourself to ride the business roller coaster up and down or to make others ride it with you. Your business will inevitably experience good times and bad ones, sometimes even in the same day, but your emotional well-being should not be tethered to them. Furthermore, part of your job as a leader is to shield your co-workers and family members from high-level uncertainties so that they can focus on what they can control and not spend needless energy worrying about the future.

Not that you should withhold important information from people who are close to you, but you must be strong enough to absorb the body blows unless it is clear that exposing others to them can help you manage through a tough situation. On the other hand, it is very important to share good news when things go well, and as I said before, use these moments as opportunities to recognize others for their contributions to it. You just need to make sure you don't ever get so high that you can't see the reality of the situation or are unprepared to deal with the next speed bump.

I wouldn't trade my mission-driven, entrepreneurial experience for anything, in spite of the speed bumps, pot holes, and a few near-death experiences. This is partially because I have been able to make a small dent in our healthcare system, achieved some financial success, worked with so many great people, and very importantly, because overcoming many challenges along the way has made me a better, stronger person, and a more effective leader. There is still plenty of work ahead to make our healthcare system more accessible and affordable, and I'm not done yet.

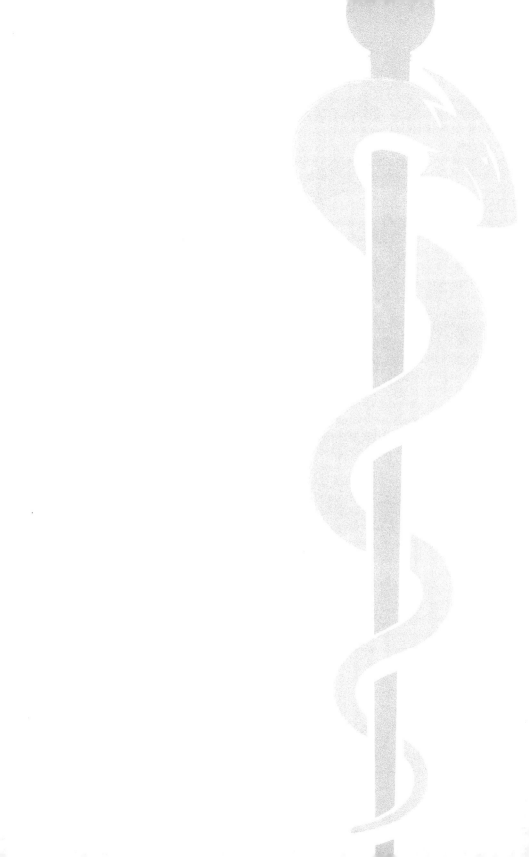

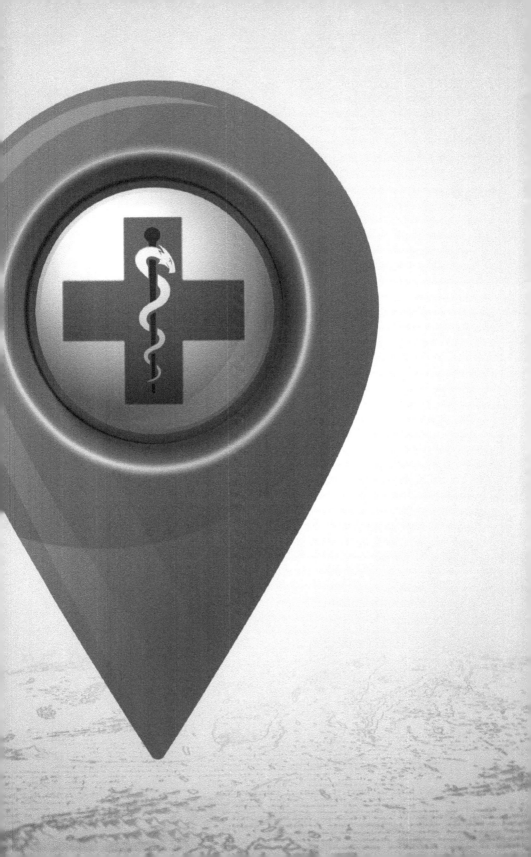

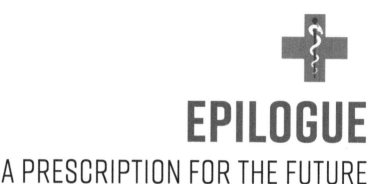

EPILOGUE
A PRESCRIPTION FOR THE FUTURE

Let me begin this epilogue by acknowledging that I am not a health policy wonk. Many people far smarter than me have tried to address the inefficiencies and inequities of our nation's healthcare system, and many of these individuals and groups have a broader perspective on the system than my more limited retail view. However, there are certain things I have observed over the course of the last thirty-five years that I strongly believe should be part of the prescription for what ails our $4 trillion healthcare system.

American Medical Communications (AMC) and America's Health Network (AHN) were innovative in their day and effective at making reliable health information more accessible to consumers. In addition, AHN.com was an early innovator in making such information inter-actively available via the internet. However, despite the fact that there are countless health-related websites today claiming to satisfy this need, it is clear that many consumers still don't know enough about how to maintain their health and well-being—or are not sufficiently motivated enough to do it—to create the degree of individual responsibility that is a necessary prerequisite for systemic success.

There are many examples of this, but the high and still rapidly growing rate of obesity in the United States—which has tripled over the past sixty years—is the most glaring of them. Today, three out of every four Americans are overweight, and more than 40 percent are clinically obese. Because of the proven connection between obesity and many debilitating and potentially deadly conditions—including diabetes, heart disease, and some cancers—the personal toll from this obesity epidemic is incalculable, and the related costs are estimated to be more than $170 billion annually.[13]

Despite our nascent efforts to address this epidemic through RediClinic's Weigh Forward program, and the existence of other well-conceived weight management programs, it is indisputable that many consumers are literally killing themselves through their sedentary lifestyles and excessive consumption of high-calorie processed foods and sugary beverages. There are many reasons for persistent growth of this deadly combination of physical inactivity and poor nutrition, but one of them is that there has been no sustained public education campaign dedicated to informing consumers about the many benefits of exercise and healthy eating, how to incorporate these things into individual and family lifestyles, and the severe consequences of ignoring them.

A similar public education campaign focused on the dangers of smoking—in combination with higher taxes on cigarettes—was

---

13   Bryan Stierman, et al., "National Health and Nutrition Examination Survey 2017–March 2020 Prepandemic Data Files Development of Files and Prevalence Estimates for Selected Health Outcomes," NHSR no. 158 (2021).

substantially responsible for cutting the incidence of smoking in the United States by almost half, from 20.9 percent in 2005 to 11.5 percent today, and it can be replicated to help reverse the seemingly inexorable obesity trend. While acknowledging that obesity has many underlying causes, a substantial and sustained public education campaign—including a strong school component—can be an important part of the solution. My view is that it should be funded, at least in part, by the food and beverage companies that are knowingly contributing to the obesity epidemic, just as the tobacco companies were forced to contribute to the smoking cessation campaign. With or without industry support, a creative, multi-media campaign that addresses the negative health and economic impacts of obesity and simple measures that individuals can take to combat it would generate a positive financial and humanistic return on whatever amount of public investment is required.

A sensitive aspect of promoting consumer health and wellness is whether third-party payors—both health insurers and employers—should be able to financially incentivize members and employees to take better care of themselves. While it is unquestionably true that some people are obese due to underlying physiologic or socioeconomic issues that are beyond their control, I have seen firsthand through the Weigh Forward program that almost everyone can lose weight and, in the process, improve their health if they have the proper support.

At the very least, third-party payors should be required to reimburse members and employees for the cost of weight management programs if they are evidence based and delivered by qualified organizations and individuals. These should include primary care physicians and other healthcare professionals, who should be trained to provide weight management counseling as a standard component of their medical education.

While empowering consumers to take responsibility for their own health is part of the solution, we also need to continue to make basic healthcare more accessible and affordable, as RediClinic and FastMed have done, and as a growing number of behavioral healthcare companies are doing. Augmenting retail-based and urgent care clinics—and primary care practices—with telemedicine will increase accessibility, as digital device integration will continue to expand the health-related services that can be provided virtually. The vision we had at both RediClinic and FastMed that patients should be treated virtually first, if possible, and then referred to a nearby clinic if necessary should be fully actualized.

Another aspect of making basic healthcare more accessible is not insisting that providers must see patients in person in order to be reimbursed for evidence-based healthcare services. My experience with Health Dialog convinced me beyond any doubt that video, digital, telephonic, and even some forms of print communication can be extremely cost-effective in helping affected individuals self-manage both acute/episodic and chronic conditions. We need to stop driving patients into healthcare facilities and spend more time and resources figuring out how to keep patients out of them unless physical contact is essential to the performance of proper diagnosis and treatment.

To make basic healthcare more accessible, we should also follow through on FastMed's vision to offer urgent and primary care at the same location. Since more than 40 percent of patients at retail-based and urgent care clinics don't have a primary care provider, we should make the handoff from the former to the latter as easy as possible through physical proximity and through electronic sharing of medical records. Conversely, primary care patients should be able to satisfy many of their urgent care needs in the same place rather than having to go to much more expensive and crowded emergency rooms when they need off-hours acute/episodic care.

A significant amount of research has shown that the lack of access to primary care is a key healthcare cost (and inequity) driver, because patients who are not receiving regular medical care frequently develop serious and expensive conditions that could have been successfully managed or avoided altogether if caught earlier. Accordingly, we should be doing everything possible to increase access and referrals to primary care and to close gaps in care by regularly checking patients' key biometric markers (blood pressure, cholesterol, hemoglobin A1C, etc.) and offering screenings and immunizations when patients seek care for acute/episodic conditions at retail-based and urgent care clinics.

In addition, to make basic healthcare more affordable, all healthcare providers must be able to practice at the top of their licenses and training. This means that highly compensated physicians shouldn't be treating conditions that APPs could treat, APPs shouldn't be treating conditions that nurses or medical assistants could treat, and so on. Third-party payors should encourage this through their contracts with providers, and both state and federal regulations must encourage it by enabling APPs, pharmacists, and other allied health professionals to expand their permitted scopes of practice without direct physician supervision when research suggests that it is safe to do so. According to some estimates, the United States will have a shortage of up to 55,000 primary care physicians by 2033,[14] so—in addition to

---

14   "AAMC Report Reinforces Mounting Physician Shortage," American Association of Medical Colleges (AAMC), June 11, 2021, https://www.aamc.org/news/press-releases/aamc-report-reinforces-mounting-physician-shortage.

incentivizing more medical students to enter primary care—we should make sure that this gap can be filled by other, less costly healthcare professionals.

As mentioned previously, our healthcare system has been slowly moving from one that reimburses providers based on the number of visits, tests and procedures to one that is based on the "value" of the care that is delivered. This transition from "volume" to "value" makes a tremendous amount of conceptual sense in primary care where providers have longitudinal relationships with patients and should be incentivized to prevent disease rather than being rewarded for treating more of it, but it has been a slow process during my multi-decade healthcare career and needs to be accelerated.

Both commercial and government payors have been picking up the pace of value-based care over the past few years. This has been most notable in Medicare, where providers under some programs are paid fixed fees ("capitated payments") for providing most of the healthcare a member requires and under other programs where they are able to share in annual savings relative to fee-for-service cost benchmarks. However, we need to finally push this approach over the top and make it the rule rather than the exception. Admittedly, there are many challenges related to creating a primarily value-based system that is fair to patients, providers, and payors alike, but the easy access to patient data that has been enabled by the most sophisticated electronic health record (EHR) systems has removed many obstacles to successful implementation.

On the subject of EHRs, the government must establish interoperability standards and strongly encourage the leading suppliers to comply with them. Our healthcare system will never become efficient without the seamless exchange of patient medical records, as this eliminates the needless and sometimes painful duplication of medical tests and results in improved outcomes because providers can easily review a patient's medical history before proceeding with diagnosis and treatment. There is some medical record sharing today through local Health Information Exchanges, and some EHRs can be configured to be interoperable, but these approaches do not go nearly far enough. Our system will continue to be fundamentally inefficient until providers are clinically integrated in this way.

Finally, we need to address the huge administrative costs related to our "free-market" approach to healthcare. While I am an entrepreneur and capitalist at heart, one of the disadvantages of having so many commercial and government payors competing against each other is that the cost of determining for each insured patient how much to collect from them at the time of service (co-pay or co-insurance payment, or the entire amount if they have not met their deductible) and of processing claims for the balances due from hundreds of third-party payors that offer literally thousands of different plans is immense. These administrative costs now represent an estimated 15–30 percent of all healthcare costs—which equates to hundreds of billions of dollars on an annual basis.[15]

To put this in perspective, U.S. spending on healthcare-related administrative costs annually accounts for twice the spending on medical care for cardiovascular disease and three times the spending for cancer care. While some administrative costs are unavoidable, it is estimated that about half of them (7.5–15 percent)—or $285–$570 billion in 2019—are wasteful.[16] These are costs that are not funding patient care, and the administrative burden of managing the revenue cycle process has gotten to the point where it is discouraging individu-

---

15   "The Role of Administrative Waste in Excess US Health Spending," Health Affairs Research Brief, October 6, 2022, DOI: 10.1377/hpb20220909.830296.

16   Ibid.

als from wanting to practice medicine in all but the largest corporate environments where there are armies of back-office employees who handle this mind-numbing but essential activity.

Without getting too far into the weeds, there are things that can be done—short of moving to a single-payor system—to reduce wasteful parts of the administrative burden, and they need to be implemented. Some of these measures revolve around simplification of the way providers are reimbursed—through the capitated structures favored by a growing number of value-based plans and by establishing case rates for the treatment of common medical conditions and bundled payments for common surgeries. Other solutions may require a degree of national centralization in the way claims are processed and providers are credentialed. Some of the administrative waste-reduction measures that have been proposed may seem antithetical to our nation's relatively free-market approach to healthcare, but compromises will need to be made to make the current system sustainable.

As I said at the beginning, this is not intended to be a comprehensive list of steps that should be taken to increase the cost-effectiveness of our nation's healthcare delivery system. These are only observations from my retail perspective and do not address parts of the system that deliver higher levels of frequently extraordinary care and beg thorny medical ethics issues—including those related to end-of-life care, which represents a significant portion of total healthcare costs, and expensive new drugs that may have marginal efficacy.

Nevertheless, addressing the areas of opportunity I have briefly described could result in meaningful improvements in the cost-effectiveness of our system and the health of those who use it. In the process, doing this would enable us to reverse the unsustainable trend in our current system, which has the unfortunate distinction of being the most expensive in the world while being one of the least effective and accessible by many of the most common measures. As I have experienced over the past thirty-five years, it is extremely difficult to effect change in this lumbering giant, but it can and must be done.

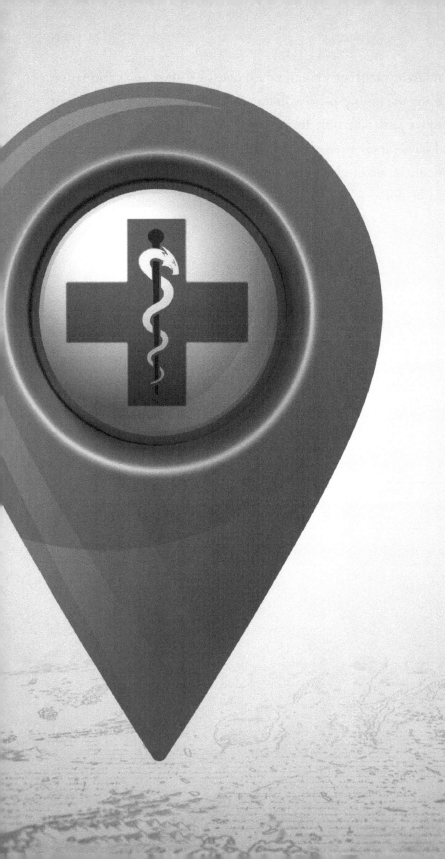

ABOUT THE AUTHOR

Web Golinkin's lifelong quest has focused on increasing the accessibility and affordability of reliable health information and basic healthcare, from America's Health Network to RediClinic, Health Dialog, and FastMed. The CEO of six companies over the past thirty-five years, he also co-founded and chaired the Convenient Care Association, has been widely covered in the national media, and has spoken at numerous healthcare conferences.

Web is a magna cum laude graduate of Harvard. He grew up in New York City and Long Island but has lived in Houston since 1988, so he is almost a Texan. A longtime marathon runner, he also enjoys tennis and golf—as long as he can walk and carry his bag. Web has been married to the same extraordinary woman for thirty-eight years, and they have two amazing sons who make him proud every day.